Exploring Disaster Human Services for Children and Youth

From Hurricane Katrina to the Paradise Wildfires

PROCEEDINGS OF A WORKSHOP SERIES

Anna Nicholson, Aurelia Attal-Juncqua, and Scott Wollek, *Rapporteurs*

Board on Health Sciences Policy

Health and Medicine Division

The National Academies of
SCIENCES · ENGINEERING · MEDICINE

THE NATIONAL ACADEMIES PRESS
Washington, DC
www.nap.edu

THE NATIONAL ACADEMIES PRESS   500 Fifth Street, NW   Washington, DC 20001

This activity was supported by a contract between the National Academy of Sciences and the Office of Human Services Emergency Preparedness and Response at the Administration for Children and Families at the Department of Health and Human Services. Any opinions, findings, conclusions, or recommendations expressed in this publication do not necessarily reflect the views of any organization or agency that provided support for the project.

International Standard Book Number-13: 978-0-309-48333-9
International Standard Book Number-10: 0-309-48333-6
Digital Object Identifier: https://doi.org/10.17226/26158

Additional copies of this publication are available from the National Academies Press, 500 Fifth Street, NW, Keck 360, Washington, DC, 20001; (800) 624-6242 or (202) 334-3313; http://www.nap.edu.

Copyright 2021 by the National Academy of Sciences. All rights reserved.

Printed in the United States of America

Suggested citation: National Academies of Sciences, Engineering, and Medicine. 2021. *Exploring disaster human services for children and youth: From Hurricane Katrina to the Paradise wildfires: Proceedings of a workshop series*. Washington, DC: The National Academies Press. https://doi.org/10.17226/26158.

The National Academies of
SCIENCES · ENGINEERING · MEDICINE

The **National Academy of Sciences** was established in 1863 by an Act of Congress, signed by President Lincoln, as a private, nongovernmental institution to advise the nation on issues related to science and technology. Members are elected by their peers for outstanding contributions to research. Dr. Marcia McNutt is president.

The **National Academy of Engineering** was established in 1964 under the charter of the National Academy of Sciences to bring the practices of engineering to advising the nation. Members are elected by their peers for extraordinary contributions to engineering. Dr. John L. Anderson is president.

The **National Academy of Medicine** (formerly the Institute of Medicine) was established in 1970 under the charter of the National Academy of Sciences to advise the nation on medical and health issues. Members are elected by their peers for distinguished contributions to medicine and health. Dr. Victor J. Dzau is president.

The three Academies work together as the **National Academies of Sciences, Engineering, and Medicine** to provide independent, objective analysis and advice to the nation and conduct other activities to solve complex problems and inform public policy decisions. The National Academies also encourage education and research, recognize outstanding contributions to knowledge, and increase public understanding in matters of science, engineering, and medicine.

Learn more about the National Academies of Sciences, Engineering, and Medicine at www.nationalacademies.org.

The National Academies of
SCIENCES • ENGINEERING • MEDICINE

Consensus Study Reports published by the National Academies of Sciences, Engineering, and Medicine document the evidence-based consensus on the study's statement of task by an authoring committee of experts. Reports typically include findings, conclusions, and recommendations based on information gathered by the committee and the committee's deliberations. Each report has been subjected to a rigorous and independent peer-review process and it represents the position of the National Academies on the statement of task.

Proceedings published by the National Academies of Sciences, Engineering, and Medicine chronicle the presentations and discussions at a workshop, symposium, or other event convened by the National Academies. The statements and opinions contained in proceedings are those of the participants and are not endorsed by other participants, the planning committee, or the National Academies.

For information about other products and activities of the National Academies, please visit www.nationalacademies.org/about/whatwedo.

PLANNING COMMITTEE ON EXPLORING BEST PRACTICES IN INTEGRATION OF PUBLIC HEALTH AND HUMAN SERVICES SERVICE DELIVERY AND ASSESSMENT FOLLOWING LARGE-SCALE DISASTERS[1]

ROBERTA LAVIN (*Chair*), Professor and Ph.D. Program Director, University of New Mexico College of Nursing
SHERLITA AMLER, Commissioner, Westchester County Department of Health
HEATHER BEAL, President and Founder, BLOCKS Inc.
ANNA FEIGUM, Emergency Services Coordinator, Oregon Department of Human Services
CAROL FLORES, Texas Disaster Case Management Program Grant Coordinator, National Voluntary Organizations Active in Disasters
JENNIFER HORNEY, Professor and Founding Director of the Program in Epidemiology and Core Faculty, University of Delaware Disaster Research Center
LESLIE LUKE, Deputy Director, Los Angeles County Office of Emergency Management
DESI MATTEL-ANDERSON, Chief Wrangler, The Field Innovation Team; Chief Executive Officer, Global Disaster Innovation Group, LLC
CHARLOTTE OLSEN, Emergency Manager, Colorado Department of Human Services
JEFF SCHLEGELMILCH, Deputy Director, National Center for Disaster Preparedness, Earth Institute, Columbia University
RICHARD SERINO, Distinguished Senior Fellow, National Preparedness Leadership Initiative, Harvard University
JOELLE SIMPSON, Medical Director for Emergency Preparedness, Children's National Hospital
TARAH SOMER, Commissioned Officer, Agency for Toxic Substances and Disease Registry (ATSDR); Regional Director, ATSDR Region 1

Health and Medicine Division Staff

SCOTT WOLLEK, Senior Program Officer
AURELIA ATTAL-JUNCQUA, Associate Program Officer
MICHAEL BERRIOS, Research Associate

---

[1] The National Academies of Sciences, Engineering, and Medicine's planning committees are solely responsible for organizing the workshop, identifying topics, and choosing speakers. The responsibility for the published Proceedings of a Workshop Series rests with the workshop rapporteurs and the institution.

KIM SUTTON, Senior Program Assistant
ANDREW M. POPE, Senior Director, Board on Health Sciences Policy

Consultants

ANNA NICHOLSON, Science Writer
LAURA RUNNELS, LAR Consulting

Reviewers

This Proceedings of a Workshop Series was reviewed in draft form by individuals chosen for their diverse perspectives and technical expertise. The purpose of this independent review is to provide candid and critical comments that will assist the National Academies of Sciences, Engineering, and Medicine in making each published proceedings as sound as possible and to ensure that it meets the institutional standards for quality, objectivity, evidence, and responsiveness to the charge. The review comments and draft manuscript remain confidential to protect the integrity of the process.

We thank the following individuals for their review of this proceedings:

GAIL KELSO, Child Care Disaster Relief and Recovery, ICF
JULIE LOOPER-COATS, ChildCare Aware of America
JESSICA VERMILYEA, Lutheran Social Services Disaster Response, Upbring

Although the reviewers listed above provided many constructive comments and suggestions, they were not asked to endorse the content of the proceedings nor did they see the final draft before its release. The review of this proceedings was overseen by **LYNN R. GOLDMAN,** Milken Institute School of Public Health, The George Washington University. She was responsible for making certain that an independent examination of this proceedings was carried out in accordance with standards of the National Academies and that all review comments were carefully considered. Responsibility for the final content rests entirely with the rapporteurs and the National Academies.

Contents

ACRONYMS AND ABBREVIATIONS		xiii
1	**INTRODUCTION**	**1**
	Workshop Objectives, 2	
	Workshop Background: Setting the Stage, 3	
	Disaster Human Services: Connecting the Human Service Networks, 4	
	Recommendations from the National Commission on Children and Disasters, 6	
	Organization of the Proceedings, 8	
	Critical Child Infrastructure, 8	
2	**EXPOSURE OUTLIERS: CHILDREN COMING OF AGE IN AN AGE OF ENVIRONMENTAL EXTREMES**	**21**
	Engaging and Learning from Children Affected by Disasters, 21	
	Cumulative Effects of Collective Trauma Events, 22	
	A Call to Action from the National Commission on Children and Disasters, 23	
	Discussion, 25	
3	**EFFECT OF DISASTERS ON CRITICAL CHILD INFRASTRUCTURE**	**29**
	Office of Child Care and the Child Care Development Fund, 29	
	Disaster Planning and Collaboration to Support Children, Youth, and Families, 33	

American Red Cross: Support for Children Across All Phases of Disasters, 34
Disaster Medicine Infrastructure Planning: Health Care System Considerations for Children, 38
Discussion, 41

4 EXPLORING THE GAPS IN EVIDENCE 45
Progress and Gaps in Supporting Children, Youth, Families, and Service Providers, 45
Study of the Effect of Hurricane Maria on Children in Puerto Rico, 48
Research Gaps in Children's Disaster Mental and Behavioral Health, 54
Discussion, 58

5 CASE STUDIES: EFFECT OF DISASTERS ON SPECIFIC POPULATIONS 65
Effect on Children with Issues Brought on by, or Exacerbated by, Disasters, 65
Effect of Disasters on Parents and Guardians, 70
Effect of Disasters on Children with Complex or Special Needs, 75
Effect of Disasters on Unaccompanied Minors, 80

6 WORKSHOP REFLECTIONS 87
Closing Reflections on the Workshop, 87
Strengthening Support for Children and Youth in Disasters, 88

REFERENCES 95

APPENDIXES

A Workshop Statement of Task 99
B Workshop Agenda 101
C Speaker Biographies 109

Boxes and Figure

BOXES

1-1 Lessons Learned from the Federal Response to Hurricane Katrina, 5

2-1 Effects of Cumulative Disaster Exposure and Prolonged Displacement, 23

3-1 Support Needs for Disaster-Affected Children, Youth, and Families, 33

4-1 Youth Development Institute of Puerto Rico, 49

FIGURE

1-1 Human-centered structured analytic approach, 9

Acronyms and Abbreviations

ACE	adverse childhood experience
ACF	Administration for Children and Families
ACL	Administration for Community Living
ANA	Administration for Native Americans
ARC	American Red Cross
ASPR	Assistant Secretary for Preparedness and Response
CARES	Coronavirus Aid, Relief, and Economic Security Act
CCDF	Child Care Development Fund
CDC	Centers for Disease Control and Prevention
COOP	continuity-of-operations plan
CPR	cardiopulmonary resuscitation
CSBG	community services block grant
EBT	electronic benefit transfer
ECD	Office of Early Childhood Development
ESF	Emergency Support Function
FEMA	Federal Emergency Management Agency
FVPSA	Family Violence Prevention and Services Act
HHS	Department of Health and Human Services
LIHEAP	Low-Income Home Energy Assistance Program

NCCD	National Commission on Children and Disasters
NCMEC	National Center for Missing & Exploited Children
OCC	Office of Child Care
OCS	Office of Community Services
OHS	Office of Head Start
OHSEPR	Office of Human Services Emergency Preparedness and Response
ORR	Office of Refugee Resettlement
OSEP	Office of Special Education Programs
OTIP	Office on Trafficking in Persons
SAMHSA	Substance Abuse and Mental Health Services Administration
SBA	Small Business Administration
SNA	social network analysis
SNAP	Supplemental Nutrition Assistance Program
SSBG	social services block grant
STC	Save the Children
TANF	Temporary Assistance for Needy Families
VOAD	voluntary organization active in disaster
WIC	Special Supplemental Nutrition Program for Women, Infants, and Children
YDI	Youth Development Institute of Puerto Rico

1

Introduction

Large-scale disasters continue to strike the United States with escalating frequency, greater magnitude, and substantial costs to the health, social, and economic welfare of affected communities (Boustan et al., 2020). From Hurricane Katrina in 2005 to the Paradise wildfires of 2018, recent disasters have exposed gaps in the capacity of the nation's critical child infrastructure (i.e., the existing systems and networks of social and human services that serve children and youth) to fully support children and youth throughout the disaster response and recovery process. Experiencing a disaster can affect the physical and emotional health of children and youth in myriad ways that extend beyond the immediate danger of physical hazards. They may face months or even years of challenging circumstances, such as displacement from their communities, interruption of their education, and disruption of regular health and social support services. Others experience the trauma of lengthy separation from their families or—particularly in the case of children and youth who are already vulnerable because of other factors—the potential for exploitation. Those who live in disaster-prone areas, such as the Gulf Coast, may experience multiple large-scale disasters before they are adults, but the effects of cumulative disaster exposure and prolonged displacement are only beginning to be understood. On the other hand, children and youth can contribute in valuable ways to bolster their families and communities throughout the recovery process. Despite their unique needs, vulnerabilities, and capabilities, children and youth have traditionally been overlooked or underconsidered in disaster planning and preparedness efforts.

WORKSHOP OBJECTIVES

To explore issues related to the effects of disasters on children and youth and lessons learned from experiences during previous disasters, the virtual workshop From Hurricane Katrina to Paradise Wildfires, Exploring Themes in Disaster Human Services was convened on July 22 and 23, 2020, by the National Academies of Sciences, Engineering, and Medicine (see Appendix A for the workshop's complete Statement of Task).[1] This workshop is the first in a series of workshops exploring promising practices, ongoing challenges, and potential opportunities that have arisen since Hurricane Katrina in the coordinated delivery of social and human services programs following federally declared major natural disasters. The workshop was sponsored by the Office of Human Services Emergency Preparedness and Response (OHSEPR) at the Administration for Children and Families (ACF) at the Department of Health and Human Services (HHS). The objectives of the workshop were the following:

- Understand the critical child infrastructure (i.e., the existing systems and networks of social and human services that serve children and youth) and how it functions (i.e., how services are delivered) before, during, and after a major federally declared natural or environmental disaster.
- Understand the negative effects of disasters on children and youth that can be mitigated by the provision of social and human services.
- Understand the current gaps and future opportunities for supporting coordinated delivery during, and restoration of services following, a major federally declared natural disaster.
- Explore potential matrices for evaluating response and recovery efforts related to social and human services.

Roberta Lavin, member of the workshop planning committee and professor at the University of New Mexico College of Nursing, detailed the intended scope of the workshop and highlighted that the past disasters discussed would span from Hurricane Katrina in 2005 to the Paradise wildfires of 2018. Lavin explained that the effects of, and the response to, the COVID-19 pandemic would not be a main point of focus during the workshop. The populations of interest were children and youth aged 0–26 years,

---

[1] The planning committee's role was limited to planning the workshop, and the Proceedings of a Workshop Series was prepared by the workshop rapporteurs as a factual summary of what occurred at the workshop. Statements, recommendations, and opinions expressed are those of individual presenters and participants, and are not necessarily endorsed or verified by the National Academies of Sciences, Engineering, and Medicine, and they should not be construed as reflecting any group consensus.

and the workshop was designed to focus on individuals who receive public support prior to disasters (i.e., people with socioeconomic deficits prior to the disaster). Additional areas of focus were the coordination of disaster response efforts and the transition to reestablishing routine service delivery programs postdisaster by human services, social services, and public health agencies at the state, local, tribal, and territorial levels. The workshop was also intended to provide a platform for highlighting promising practices, ongoing challenges, and potential opportunities for coordinated delivery and restoration of social and human services programs.

WORKSHOP BACKGROUND: SETTING THE STAGE

Scott Lekan, principal deputy assistant secretary at ACF, described the rationale for the workshop and reviewed ACF's goals during and after disasters. In his capacity as principal deputy assistant, he supports the management and daily operations of 64 programs and 16 program offices within ACF designed to support individuals, families, and communities in crisis. ACF is the largest grant maker within HHS, providing approximately $8 billion annually through direct funding to households and other grantees. These funds are intended to provide communities with the necessary services to support their economic resilience and develop individuals by centering their life experience in human service delivery models. ACF's programs support a wide range of human and social services, including early childhood education, support for abused and neglected children, support for trafficked persons and survivors of domestic violence, temporary financial assistance, and job training and education. He noted that the workshop's participants included an array of thought leaders in emergency management and disaster operations who have special expertise in issues affecting children and youth in postdisaster contexts.

Lekan emphasized that children are not merely small adults; they require tailored support because disasters or other traumas can affect children's development. After a disaster, affected communities—particularly vulnerable groups and children—need appropriately targeted support. To identify a path forward in the face of increasingly complex and layered disasters, ACF is focused on childhood adoption, primary prevention, and promoting person-centered, whole family–integrated, streamlined services by moving from a compliance delivery model to one focused on measuring outcomes. ACF works across federal agencies such as the Department of Housing and Urban Development, the Department of Education, and other HHS agencies such as the Substance Abuse and Mental Health Services Administration (SAMHSA) and the Administration for Community Living (ACL). He added that while ACF's overarching aim is primary prevention, it also focuses on supporting communities through child care systems that enable people to work while safely supporting their children's development. Lekan explained that helping individuals return to work after disasters is necessary for communities to begin recovering economically. He encouraged workshop participants to incorporate the messages that emerge from the workshop into their ongoing disaster readiness efforts as well, as ACF plans to do.

DISASTER HUMAN SERVICES: CONNECTING THE HUMAN SERVICE NETWORKS

Natalie Grant, director of OHSEPR at ACF, described the genesis of federal disaster human services and how they are situated within the broader human services networks today. ACF promotes the economic and social well-being of families, children, individuals, and communities. Each ACF office has a director or a commissioner who ensures that the activities of the office support ACF's mission. She likened social and human services delivery to a patchwork quilt, suggesting that the various social and human services that affect the lives of individuals must be pieced together, especially when responding to disasters. The recognition that these services must be connected led to the creation of OHSEPR in 2006.

Grant explained that in 2006, a report by the Executive Office of the President on the federal response to Hurricane Katrina found that a major challenge in the delivery of human services was the disconnected network of independent actors, programs, and services that were not adequately coordinated to meet the needs of the disaster survivors (DHS, 2006) (see Box 1-1). In 2006, the White House responded by issuing a directive that HHS coordinate with other departments of the executive branch, state governments, and nongovernmental organizations to develop a robust, comprehensive, and integrated system to deliver services during disasters. In addition to ACF being tasked by HHS to coordinate with other HHS operating divisions to develop this capacity, another outcome of the directive was the creation of OHSEPR to provide policy development, coordination, guidance, and support to the ACF assistant secretary and ACF regional offices. The focus of OHSEPR is to coordinate ACF programs in partnership with other social and human service providers (e.g., SAMHSA, the Health Resources and Services Administration, the Centers for Medicare & Medicaid Services, and ACL). She noted that all of those entities have programs and touch points with the lived experience and that those social and human services were designed to help facilitate this type of coordination after a disaster.

> **BOX 1-1**
> **Lessons Learned from the**
> **Federal Response to Hurricane Katrina**
>
> - Federal preparation for distributing individual assistance proved frustrating and inadequate.
> - Because the National Response Plan did not mandate a single federal point of contact for all assistance and required the Federal Emergency Management Agency to merely coordinate assistance delivery, disaster victims confronted an enormously bureaucratic, inefficient, and frustrating process that failed to effectively meet their needs.
> - The federal government's system for distribution of human services was not sufficiently responsive to the circumstances of a large number of victims—many of whom were particularly vulnerable—who were forced to navigate a series of complex processes to obtain critical services in a time of extreme duress.
>
> SOURCES: Grant presentation, July 22, 2020; DHS, 2006.

Grant described how ACF's programs fit into the broader disaster response network through their focus on:

- Integrated and holistic service delivery through community hubs,
- Family-focused case management empowered by digital platforms,
- Flexible policies and programs that foster innovation such as disaster waivers and flexibilities,[2] and
- A crisis management approach to changing human service delivery.

Grant added that OHSEPR has also established three national priorities to build a coordinated national disaster human services capability. The first priority is to develop "disaster human services" as an ACF-led HHS enterprise. The second is to develop effective partnerships to execute the department's mission for health and human services as part of the Federal Emergency Management Agency's (FEMA's) Emergency Support Function (ESF) 6.[3] The third is to maintain focus by developing outcome-oriented solutions, reducing the burden to jurisdictions through collaboration, and demonstrating the value proposition to engaged parties.

---

[2] More information about ACF disaster waivers and flexibilities is available at https://www.acf.hhs.gov/ohsepr/training-technical-assistance/acf-emergency-and-disaster-waivers-and-flexibilities (accessed May 20, 2021).

[3] More information about FEMA's ESF 6 is available at https://www.fema.gov/pdf/emergency/nrf/nrf-esf-06.pdf (accessed March 2, 2021).

Grant provided an overview of ACF–OHSEPR roles in leadership, coordination, and partnership, noting that ACF activities are nested within the ecosystem of HHS programs, federal interagency activities, and the activities of national and nongovernmental partners. OHSEPR coordinates disaster human services by leading disaster human service delivery and coordination, developing ESF 6 and ESF 8,[4] and partnering with HHS operation divisions and staff divisions on operational planning aspects of ESF 6. Grant noted that the office learned from previous disaster experiences and is

- developing jurisdictional emergency management human service capability;
- connecting health care, public health, and human services to create partnerships;
- partnering with HHS operation divisions and other federal emergency management components on predisaster readiness; and
- developing the disaster human services science agenda.

Regarding the latter, she explained that the goal is to initiate the development of a body of evidence-based knowledge for disaster human services. The focus is on identifying substantive observations, significant changes, and ongoing deficits in disaster human services provision and coordination that have occurred since Hurricane Katrina. The desired outcome is the development of a roadmap for providing timely, coordinated, and appropriately targeted human services after disasters. She noted that the workshop on children and youth in disasters was convened to help move the field of disaster science forward, with future workshops planned to explore population displacement in disasters as well as data sharing and information management in disaster human services.

RECOMMENDATIONS FROM THE NATIONAL COMMISSION ON CHILDREN AND DISASTERS

To further help contextualize the workshop's objectives, Lavin highlighted several recommendations made by the National Commission on Children and Disasters in its 2010 report to the president and Congress (NCCD and AHRQ, 2010). She assessed the current status and progress toward achieving those recommendations and highlighted areas where further work is needed.

Recommendation 2.3 called for federal agencies and nonfederal partners to enhance predisaster preparedness and just-in-time training in pediatric

---

[4] More information about FEMA's ESF 8 is available at https://www.fema.gov/sites/default/files/2020-07/fema_ESF_8_Public-Health-Medical.pdf (accessed March 2, 2021).

disaster mental and behavioral health—including psychological first aid, bereavement support, and brief supportive interventions—for mental health professionals and individuals, such as teachers, who work with children. Lavin said that psychological first aid has been successfully implemented and is now being taught nationwide, with organizations like the Children's Bereavement Center of South Texas working with organizations such as FEMA and the American Red Cross to provide support after disasters.

Recommendation 5.2 called for disaster case management programs to be appropriately resourced and to provide consistent holistic services that achieve tangible, positive outcomes for children and families affected by the disaster. ACF has operated a disaster case management program for more than 10 years, Lavin noted. Recommendation 6.1 called for Congress and federal agencies to improve disaster preparedness capabilities for child care. After Hurricane Sandy, it became a requirement that child care providers have disaster plans. Recommendation 6.2 called for Congress and federal agencies to improve capacity to provide child care services in the immediate aftermath of and recovery from disasters, including codifying child care as an essential service of a governmental nature. Lavin noted that some states have since designated child care as an essential service, including New York. Recommendation 6.3 called for HHS to require disaster preparedness capabilities for Head Start centers and basic disaster mental health training for staff. In 2009, Head Start published the *Head Start Emergency Preparedness Manual*, which has since been updated and includes many resources.[5] Furthermore, FEMA has since published an emergency preparedness guide for Head Start.[6]

Lavin said that despite this progress, there is room for improvement. For instance, Recommendation 7.1 calls for ensuring that school systems recovering from disasters are provided with immediate resources to reopen and restore the learning environment in a timely manner and provide support for displaced students and their host schools, including funding. Additionally, Recommendation 8.2 calls for ensuring that state and local juvenile justice agencies and all residential treatment, correctional, and detention facilities that house children can adequately prepare for disasters. She pointed out that the Cybersecurity and Infrastructure Security Agency does not list child care, schools, and human services as critical infrastructure sectors; she proposed that these three sectors be classified as critical infrastructure sectors.[7]

---

[5] More information about the FEMA Preparedness Portal is available at https://community.fema.gov/AP_Login?startURL=%2Fstory%2Femergency-preparedness-for-head-start%3Flang%3Den_us (accessed October 26, 2020).

[6] More information about the *Head Start Emergency Preparedness Manual* is available at https://rems.ed.gov/docs/Head_Start_Emergency_Preparedness_Manual.pdf (accessed October 26, 2020).

[7] More information about critical infrastructure sectors is available at https://www.cisa.gov/critical-infrastructure-sectors (accessed October 26, 2020).

To establish a path forward, Lavin suggested applying a human-centered structured analytic approach (see Figure 1-1). This approach puts children as the end users and requires exploration through empathizing using ethnography; assessing local, state, and federal regulations; and identifying the scope of practice by states and territories. However, Lavin explained that the scope of human services will need to be better specified in order to identify the evidence base needed to optimize this approach; stakeholder meetings, such as the present workshop, can contribute to developing that evidence base and establishing actionable items. She added that new approaches should address the issues of flexibility, speed, and support to states, as well as self-determination, self-sufficiency, and federalism.

ORGANIZATION OF THE PROCEEDINGS

This Proceedings of a Workshop Series is organized into six chapters. The second half of Chapter 1 focuses on providing an overview of critical child infrastructure and the framework of disaster response services for children. Chapter 2 summarizes the workshop's keynote address, which explores the effects of environmental extremes on children and disasters. Chapter 3 focuses on the effects of disasters on critical child infrastructure. Chapter 4 explores the gaps in evidence relating to children in disasters. Chapter 5 presents case studies from four breakout panels held during the workshop, which focused on the effect on children with issues brought on by, or exacerbated by, disasters; the effect of disasters on parents and guardians; the effect of disasters on children with complex or special needs; and the effect of disasters on unaccompanied minors. Chapter 6 presents the reflections of workshop participants and speakers and explores ways to pursue the outcomes and objectives set forth by the workshop.

CRITICAL CHILD INFRASTRUCTURE

The first panel of the workshop provided an overview of critical child infrastructure and the framework of disaster response services for children. The session's aims were (1) to review existing systems and networks of social and human services that help children, review how these services are delivered in normal times, and review how these services prepare for major federally declared disasters; and (2) to identify flaws and gaps in the normal delivery of services that become more harmful when disasters strike. The session was moderated by Tarah Somers, regional director, Region 1 of the Agency for Toxic Substances and Disease Registry.

INTRODUCTION

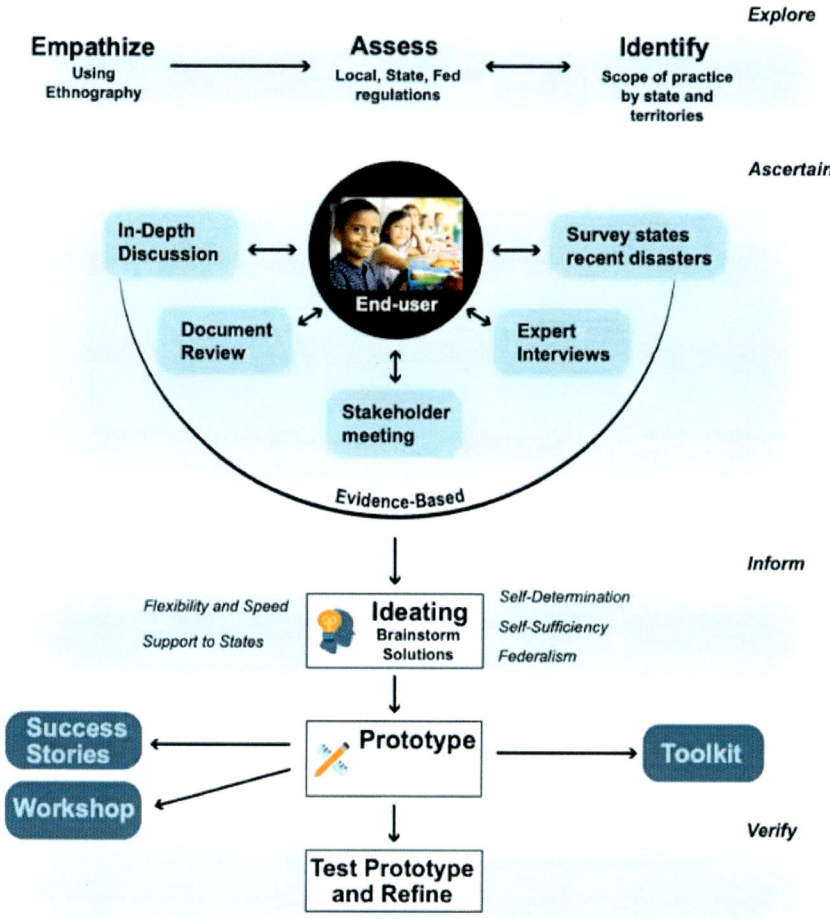

FIGURE 1-1 Human-centered structured analytic approach.
SOURCE: Lavin presentation, July 23, 2020.

Administration for Children and Families and Steady-State Preparation for Natural Disasters[8]

Deborah Bergeron, director of the Office of Head Start (OHS) and director of the Office of Early Childhood Development at ACF, discussed

---

[8] This section is based on the presentation of Deborah Bergeron, director of OHS and director of the Office of Early Childhood Development at ACF.

steady-state[9] preparation for natural disasters. She outlined the efforts of ACF offices to provide emergency assistance, domestic violence prevention, homeless youth services, disaster preparation for Native American and tribal communities, human trafficking prevention, refugee resettlement, and child welfare services. She noted that one of the Office of Early Childhood Development's goals is to bring early childhood issues to the table throughout ACF and find common areas where offices can collaborate to be more efficient and effective in serving children during disasters.

Office of Community Services/Office of Family Assistance

The Low-Income Home Energy Assistance Program (LIHEAP) is run by the Office of Community Services (OCS)/Office of Family Assistance. The program provides funding to states, territories, and tribes to assist with home energy bills for low-income households. Bergeron noted that while the program's focus is on heating and cooling—through bill payment assistance and weatherization services—LIHEAP funding can also be used to respond to disasters. This can include temporary housing, transportation to shelters, generators, energy-related home repairs, and other specified emergency needs. LIHEAP assistance is available for both temporary disasters and long-term events.

Family Youth Services Bureau

The Family Youth Service Bureau addresses needs related to family violence and homeless youth during a disaster. The Family Violence Prevention and Services Act (FVPSA) provides funding for emergency shelter and other supportive services to domestic violence victims and their children. Bergeron noted that domestic violence tends to increase during disasters owing to heightened stress caused by these events, thus disaster preparedness and domestic violence prevention are related. To ensure collaboration, an FVPSA liaison works with the OHSEPR team in this effort. The Family Youth Services Bureau also addresses the needs of children via its Runaway and Homeless Youth unit. This program has an emergency preparedness plan that includes strategies for addressing evacuation, food insecurity, medical supplies, and notification of youths' families, when appropriate. A challenge that this unit faces is that children who are not linked with a home can be difficult to locate, she added.

---

[9] "Steady-state" refers to normal operations, when no incident or specific risk or hazard has been identified.

Administration for Native Americans

The Administration for Native Americans (ANA) focuses on disaster preparation for Native American and tribal communities. Training is the focus of ANA's national disaster preparation, said Bergeron. ANA provides resources on natural disaster preparation on its website—which also provides disaster preparedness resources—and through webinar trainings and in-person training opportunities. In February 2020, ACF hosted a large Native American grantee meeting that included training from OHSEPR on disaster preparedness, such as planning in advance for service provision and developing continuity-of-operations plans. Bergeron noted that the meeting was held before the COVID-19 pandemic was recognized in the United States and was reflective of ANA's steady state of affairs.

Office on Trafficking in Persons

Working closely with OHSEPR and the Office of the Assistant Secretary for Preparedness and Response (ASPR), the Office on Trafficking in Persons (OTIP) identified flexibilities and waivers for grantees and developed an infographic titled "Preventing Human Trafficking: What Disaster Responders Need to Do."[10] OTIP raises awareness that disasters increase the risk of human trafficking and provides guidance on disaster-related readiness, response, and recovery steps, said Bergeron. The office also conducted a literature review on human trafficking and natural disasters to inform public awareness efforts as well as program and policy development. The flexibilities identified by OTIP include administrative relief in the form of postponing deadlines for submission of program performance and financial reports, as well as the option to extend client enrollment in federal antitrafficking programs administered by OTIP during a natural disaster. Bergeron highlighted the importance of flexibilities in responding to disasters, noting that the state of emergency in the United States related to the COVID-19 pandemic further underscores the extent to which flexibility is important.

Office of Refugee Resettlement

Policy flexibilities during natural disasters are also a focus of the Office of Refugee Resettlement (ORR), said Bergeron. For example, in 2017, ORR issued policy letter 17-03, which provided funding and waiver opportuni-

---

[10] More information about preventing human trafficking is available at https://www.phe.gov/Preparedness/planning/abc/Documents/disaster-resp-trafficking.pdf (accessed October 27, 2020).

ties after Hurricanes Harvey and Irma.[11] She noted that these types of policy flexibilities are typically designed for events such as hurricanes and blizzards; thus, during a global pandemic, determinations have to be made as to whether these flexibilities apply. To support unaccompanied youth, ORR's Unaccompanied Alien Children program partnered with ASPR, OHSEPR, and ACF's Division of Planning and Logistics to monitor threats, report effects to care providers, and provide necessary follow-up actions. The Division of Planning and Logistics also provides training to Unaccompanied Alien Children program divisions on emergency preparedness and response throughout the year to ensure that staff are trained and prepared for potential natural disasters. She added that both OHS and ORR are concerned with the needs of children in the care of other organizations and how these children will respond to a disaster or emergency.

Children's Bureau

The Children's Bureau section of the Social Security Act, section 422(b)(16),[12] requires state child welfare agencies to have disaster preparedness plans in place. These state plans must describe how a state would do the following:

- Identify, locate, and continue the availability of services for children under state care who are affected by a disaster.
- Respond appropriately to new child welfare cases in disaster areas.
- Remain in communication with child welfare personnel displaced by a disaster.
- Preserve essential program records.
- Coordinate services and share information with other states.

Bergeron remarked that both coordination of services and communication are critical when disasters displace people and cut them off from normal lines of communication.

Office of Head Start

To prepare for natural disasters, OHS coordinates with other child welfare offices on the ground and has developed its own emergency pre-

---

[11] More information about ORR's policies on populations displaced or affected by Hurricanes Harvey or Irma is available at https://www.acf.hhs.gov/orr/resource/orr-populations-displaced-or-affected-by-hurricanes-harvey-and-irma (accessed October 27, 2020).

[12] More information about the Social Security Act, section 422(b)(16), is available at https://www.ssa.gov/OP_Home/ssact/title04/0422.htm (accessed October 27, 2020).

paredness manual.[13] Bergeron stated that OHS also provides strong support to its grantees and programs to create their own setting-specific plans tailored to the types of natural disasters more common in a given area; such plans include establishing family engagement systems and embedding mental health systems. She explained that OHS directs federal funding to local grantees running Head Start programs and is responsible for oversight of those programs. Flexible language is also in place to enable OHS to mobilize when disasters occur. For example, the response by OHS to the COVID-19 pandemic used policy language developed during Hurricane Maria. She noted that the most vulnerable children and families are affected when disasters displace entire communities. Disaster situations give rise to immediate needs (e.g., food) as well as to long-term needs such as mental health supports. Furthermore, once a program is rebuilt and reopens, the children return having experienced trauma. In Puerto Rico, for instance, when programs reopened after Hurricane Maria, teachers noticed that some children would panic when the weather shifted because of associations with the hurricane. Therefore, they try to "front load" support for such situations rather than being reactionary, she added.

Systems and Services to Support Children and Families During Disasters[14]

Josephine Bias-Robinson, board member at Life Pieces to Masterpieces, provided an overview of the disaster response programs in OCS and how they interrelate. She discussed federal, state, and local organizations with which OCS partners in disaster response, recovery, and revitalization efforts, as well as outlining OCS's role in providing guidance and clarification on eligibility status and funding flexibilities during crisis assistance and recovery.

Office of Community Services

The mission of OCS is to increase the capacity of individuals and families to become more self-sufficient and to help build, revitalize, and strengthen their communities. Bias-Robinson noted that discussions of children and youth cannot be separated from discussions of families. Thus, OCS provides opportunities to directly affect hundreds of thousands of people through the office's programs as well as connecting the federal level to local communities.

---

[13] The OHS *Emergency Preparedness Manual* is available at https://eclkc.ohs.acf.hhs.gov/sites/default/files/pdf/emergency-preparedness-manual-early-childhood-programs.pdf (accessed October 28, 2020).

[14] This section is based on the presentation of Josephine Bias-Robinson, board member at Life Pieces to Masterpieces.

Bias-Robinson explained that block grants are OCS's primary programs; they push funds, resources, and information into communities. For instance, the social services block grant (SSBG), community services block grant (CSBG), and LIHEAP provide funding directly to states. These programs also provide opportunities for states to coordinate on a localized level with community partners. By providing the bulk of human services federal funding that flows into states, these block grants direct funds to community action agencies via state social services, human resources, and labor departments. The block grants also provide flexibility in terms of the types of community services they fund. She noted that these block grants are the vehicles for supplemental funding to be distributed to states when disaster strikes. The nature of these programs and the legislative authorities they have within states lend themselves to use in times of disaster, she added. For example, in the response to Hurricane Katrina, the SSBG was one of the first vehicles that Congress used to authorize supplemental funding to states, including Texas and some of the outlying states that received evacuees.

Bias-Robinson outlined additional OCS programs that are secondary in disaster response, providing mechanisms to deliver disaster response services if funding is available and can be repurposed or amplified. These include Assets for Independence, Urban and Rural and Community Economic Development, and additional programs that were available after Hurricane Katrina but are no longer funded as part of OCS (e.g., the Community Food and Nutrition program, the Compassion Capital Fund, the Job Opportunities for Low-Income Individuals program, and the Rural Facilities Program). Although these latter programs were no longer funded at the time of the workshop, Bias-Robinson said that they were valuable in supporting affected communities during times of disaster.

Partnerships to Support Response, Recovery, and Revitalization

Bias-Robinson emphasized that "we are in this together." OCS's principal goal is to help during times of crisis by meeting emergency needs and assisting in recovery; this goal is shared with other ACF offices and across the federal government. She described this as an inherent component of OCS's history and of the tradition of community action agencies. State and local agencies that received OCS funding, particularly community action agencies, provided critical frontline communication, coordination, services, and support to low-income children and families in communities devastated and dislocated by Hurricanes Katrina and Rita. In her own experiences during those hurricanes, community action agencies were on the frontlines. Connected at the local level and working in partnership with nonprofit organizations, community action agencies are equipped with knowledge of the specific needs in their communities. She said these agencies were an on-the-ground asset that enabled OCS to have direct communication at the local level, which can be a challenge for federal agencies. Bias-Robinson said that they relied on regional administrators and ACF's Office of Regional Operations to channel communication from frontline community action agencies to OCS.

Bias-Robinson remarked that in addition to community action agencies, OCS partners with many other organizations in responding to disasters, during which coordination and communication with all available partners is vital. These include state departments of human services, health and welfare, and economic opportunity, as well as corresponding regional offices. Large nonprofit organizations, such as the American Red Cross and the United Way, are partners in disaster response. Bias-Robinson said faith-based and community-based organizations (e.g., shelters, food banks, civic organizations) often step in quickly to respond to disasters.[15] Departments of education, local schools, and recreation centers also partner in disaster response. For example, during the September 11, 2001, terrorist attacks, Bias-Robinson worked in the White House and coordinated with local District of Columbia schools to shelter children in bomb shelters located in many school buildings. She added that other federal entities, such as the Departments of Housing and Urban Development, Labor, Transportation, and Agriculture, coordinate with ACF regional administrators and HHS regional health administrators to provide disaster relief services.

Provision of Guidance, Clarification, and Flexibility for Recovery

In determining the "who, what, why, when, and how" of the overall government response to disaster, Bias-Robinson said that providing guidance and assisting in eligibility determinations are important OCS roles. In times of disaster, people experience multiple losses, such as losing their homes, access to important documentation and paperwork, and connections. OCS provides guidance to states for determining eligibility of affected individuals and for identifying allowable services and supports funded by SSBGs, CSBGs, and LIHEAP. Furthermore, OCS shares possible strategies for community action assistance to low-income individuals and families during the initial phases of relief and recovery. Identifying flexibilities and available sources of support for expanded community action service expedites access to support for individuals and families, Bergeron stated. For example, OCS helps states ascertain expenses allowable via LIHEAP and issues waivers for the purpose of making resources more readily accessible

---

[15] Bias-Robinson noted that OCS once operated the Compassion Capital Fund to build the capacity of these small organizations.

to communities. This can apply to both the communities directly affected by disaster as well as to communities receiving displaced individuals. After Hurricanes Katrina and Rita, some states that received a smaller number of evacuees, such as Nebraska, did not have the same resources as states like Texas with large numbers of evacuees. OCS worked with states like Nebraska to identify resources, clarify how to access these resources, provide strategies on how to assist families in the initial phases of disaster relief with needs such as temporary housing, and ultimately how to support families in relocation and rebuilding. She added that OCS encourages essential community action communication and coordination with key public and private emergency responders and service providers at all phases of crisis assistance and recovery.

Discussion

Collaboration with Local Organizations

A participant asked how ACF currently shares resources and education with local emergency planners and social services organizations. Bergeron said that from the standpoint of OHS, community action agencies are important partners on the ground. Many of these agencies are Head Start grantees that partner directly with others providing services at disaster sites. Therefore, ACF's information resources often flow to other organizations via community action agencies. Bergeron said that the Head Start program is designed to partner local Head Start agencies with community organizations, which is included in OHS requirements and creates a network that provides support.

Social Services Block Grant Use During Disasters

Another participant noted that SSBGs were used in response to Hurricane Sandy and asked whether use of SSBGs in response to a disaster is an exception or considered best practice. Bias-Robinson responded that states outline their plans for how they intend to spend SSBG funds. Because there is a Child Care Bureau,[16] large funding from the bureau is prioritized. In times of supplemental funding, she said there might be opportunities to use SSBGs in this way, but states determine what is needed at that point in time.

---

[16] The Child Care Bureau was renamed the Office of Child Care in September 2010.

Features of Effective Steady-State Systems

Somers asked about features of systems that function successfully during normal times before a disaster strikes. Bergeron responded that best practices during normal times result from the learning that takes place during a disaster. As each disaster provides different challenges, each brings opportunities for learning that can be applied in addressing future disasters. She said that the objective is to be as prepared as possible to respond to disaster in a proactive, thoughtful way, rather than taking a reactive approach. Bergeron noted that the 2018 California Camp Fire disaster devastated communities and Head Start agencies, with both similarities and differences to the devastation in Puerto Rico from Hurricane Maria. She said that reflecting and growing from each type of disaster enables ACF to be even more prepared for the future.

Bias-Robinson emphasized the value of knowledge within an organization. She cited the strong OCS knowledge base during Hurricanes Katrina and Rita, built from the experiences of individuals who had served for a long period of time, seen a number of disasters, and had learned from those events. "While every disaster is unique, we do not have to recreate the wheel every single time," she said. Clear coordination, guidance, access to information, and decision making are what are needed from government offices during disasters. She added that time is lost when people are not informed, so when an agency has information, it needs to take action.

Bergeron provided the recent example of OHS's response to the COVID-19 pandemic. In March 2020, Head Start programs began shutting down nationwide for an undetermined duration. Bergeron said that her immediate concern was the 250,000 Head Start employees who needed to be paid. Even though the doors of centers were closed, Head Start continued providing services, and she wanted to ensure that employees continued to be compensated. As an example of how preparation from previous disasters allows for prompt support, she described how OHS used flexibilities that were implemented in Puerto Rico after Hurricane Maria that allowed for a nimble, quick response that prevented anyone from missing a paycheck, she said.

Effect of Disaster-Related Trauma on Children

Lavin stated that in her previous work at ACF and in emergency preparedness, she has learned that children are more significantly affected and at greater risk during a disaster than adults. She asked what ACF, private organizations, or faith-based organizations have done to ensure that children's needs are met during a disaster and to tailor services to this population. Bergeron replied that addressing trauma and adverse childhood experiences (ACEs)[17] is built into the Head Start program. She said that while disasters can be an obvious source of adverse effects on children, most Head Start programs serve children experiencing less visible underlying issues on an ongoing basis. Therefore, the trauma-informed care that OHS incorporates into its regular programming better prepares it for this aspect of disasters. Bergeron noted the trend in K–12 education of providing professional development on trauma-informed care to entire teams of staff rather than solely to professionals with mental health training. She said this trend better prepares education professionals to identify and appropriately respond to signs of trauma in children.

Agreeing that the child response to disaster looks different than the adult response, Bergeron said that sometimes children express themselves in ways that may require paying close attention to understand. In an example of Puerto Rican students responding to thunderstorms, she noted that child care workers had to be aware that when children had a hard time during storms, it was because they were associating thunderstorms with the horrible experience of a hurricane and they could not yet separate it from more mild weather events. Bergeron said having resources on hand enables organizations to respond swiftly, which she sees as a focus of all ACF programs that deal directly with children. Furthermore, in the general community, there is typically a greater connection to mental health services for both children and adults. She noted that in the past few months of the COVID-19 pandemic, there have been creative uses of technology and tele–mental health outreach, which is a way to stay connected with children and make sure that they are taken care of.

Multilevel Collaborations in Child Services

Somers asked for specific examples of youth and children services provided via successful collaborations at the federal, state, and local levels. Bias-Robinson cited her experience as chief of engagement for the District of Columbia Public Schools and the role of schools in responding to disaster. She said the school system worked directly with the mayor and in consultation with others in the region to determine a response, and they communicated the status of children to the mayor. School systems can play a critical role as a first point of dissemination by communicating to children through their parents and via other networks. She added that including schools is critically important to the disaster recovery process. Schools can be used as communication channels, and many children and families receive services through schools, including health and mental health services in

---

[17] More information about ACEs is available at https://www.cdc.gov/violenceprevention/acestudy/index.html (accessed October 23, 2020).

some cases. In the response to COVID-19, Bias-Robinson said she has been consulting with schools in the District of Columbia and Maryland to help them remain connected to their families, as this is the basis and foundation of how families receive information and support. Often, families trust their schools and school leaders to deliver these services, she concluded.

Bergeron said the message of the importance of schools cannot be overemphasized. Going where affected people are is the "whole point" of disaster services, and schools are where people are. She said that OHS has made efforts to better align early education—predominantly via Head Start—with school systems to create one response stream rather than separate, siloed responses for children younger than 5 years and those older than 5 years. Bergeron stated that better alignment would improve the effectiveness of responses to children in disasters.

Incorporating Adverse Childhood Events into Disaster Response Systems

A participant asked how the ACE framework has affected ACF's infrastructure and systems design for addressing the needs of children and youth before, during, and after natural disasters. Bergeron said that a recent example is the listing of trauma-informed care in OHS funding for quality improvements, indicating that resources need to be designated specifically for that purpose. She said trauma-informed care applies before, during, and after a disaster. Programs aligned with ACEs and that train their staff are programmatically prepared for dealing with the trauma of disaster. She said that she is not able to speak specifically about other offices' particular approaches to ACEs, but in general, there is a better understanding of the effect of trauma on brain development and on the importance of funneling resources toward mitigating those effects. This includes specific approaches with proven outcomes that enable professionals to be more responsive. From her experience in education, Bergeron said teachers often do not have a repertoire of trauma training; thus, many people interacting with children need that support. She therefore concluded that preparation is not solely about the child, but rather about the entire operation.

2

Exposure Outliers: Children Coming of Age in an Age of Environmental Extremes

Lori Peek, director of the Natural Hazards Center and professor at the University of Colorado Boulder, delivered the keynote address. She described the landscape of increased disasters, crises, and threats currently experienced by children and youth in the United States and explained how cumulative disaster exposure can have negative effects on survivors. She also called for placing the perspectives of children and youth in the center of the effort to improve disaster response services. Peek defined cumulative disaster exposure and outlined its negative effects on survivors. Roberta Lavin, professor at the University of New Mexico College of Nursing, moderated the session.

ENGAGING AND LEARNING FROM CHILDREN AFFECTED BY DISASTERS

Peek remarked that the current generation of children is coming of age in a world that is drier and hotter than ever before, is regularly punctuated by severe storms, and will almost certainly continue to be ravaged by climate extremes. Peek stated that as of July 2020, the COVID-19 pandemic claimed more than 600,000 lives globally and upended billions more; the United States continued to be convulsed by protests against racism and other forms of inequality; and the epidemic of gun violence continued to devastate young lives. She added that March 2020 was the first month of March in nearly two decades without a school shooting in the United States. Children and youth of this generation know no other world than one marked by disaster, she said, noting that this is especially true for those in low-income areas and in communities of color—populations that almost always "suffer first and worst" in this age of extremes. Having so many children living in a permanent state of emergency in the United States has stirred the collective conscience and the intellectual imagination of those participating in research and practice related to children and disasters. She maintained that although there is cause for great concern, there is also hope that can be gleaned from children and youth. Peek said that it is vital to engage children and youth, listen to what they have to say, and learn from the impressive actions that they are already taking in response to the threats of natural hazards. For this reason, she called for a follow up to the 2010 National Commission on Children and Disasters (NCCD) that is child and youth led.

Peek said that in the 15 years she has spent working with and learning from children and the adults who parent, teach, coach, treat, and support them, she has developed a deep and abiding respect for the knowledge of children. She suggested that the stories of the intellectual creativity, moral courage, and compassion that these children and their caregivers have shown during times of great loss and suffering should be captured and used for systematic learning and, ultimately, for the improvement of service provision during times of disaster. To that end, Peek has documented stories of child survivors of Hurricane Katrina in two multiyear ethnographic projects. She and Alice Fothergill of the Department of Sociology at The University of Vermont co-authored the book *Children of Katrina* (Fothergill and Peek, 2015). Peek also edited and contributed to *Displaced: Life in the Katrina Diaspora*, a collection of scholarly accounts of the resettlement experiences of mostly African American Katrina survivors who were scattered across the nation following the storm (Weber and Peek, 2014).

CUMULATIVE EFFECTS OF COLLECTIVE TRAUMA EVENTS

Peek described how cumulative effects of collective trauma events can affect people in myriad ways. From 2005 to 2015, the U.S. Gulf Coast experienced numerous disasters, with more than a dozen major disaster declarations in the State of Louisiana alone. Beginning with the catastrophic Hurricanes Katrina and Rita in 2005, the decade brought Hurricanes Gustav and Ike in 2008, the *Deepwater Horizon* oil spill in 2010, Hurricane Isaac in 2012, and additional severe storms and flooding. These events caused billions of dollars in damages, destroyed millions of homes, schools, and businesses, and upended countless lives. Although many different measures are used in social and behavioral sciences to assess the human toll of disasters, said Peek, the words of children demonstrate the impact that a successive shock of disasters can have on young people. For example, she interviewed an African American teen who was 6 years old at the time of

Hurricane Katrina. When asked at age 17 what it was like to grow up in the context of so many disasters, he said, "What I thought was a childhood was just me really preparing myself for the next natural disaster to come."

Peek defined cumulative disaster exposure as "multiple, acute onset, large-scale collective events that cause disruptions for individuals, families, and entire communities" (Mohammad and Peek, 2019). She stated that those who have experienced three or more major, community-level disasters that have had a substantial effect on both the individual and their household during their first 18 years of life are considered "exposure outliers." These youth are statistical outliers because their multiple experiences with disaster are not normative. However, Peek surmised that those norms may change given the increasing frequency of disasters, and that in an increasingly turbulent and unequal world, researchers should seek to learn more about the cumulative effects of collective trauma from children who are exposure outliers. Drawing on the limited research available on cumulative effects of disasters and the more robust literature on adverse childhood experiences at the individual level, Peek outlined a number of ways that cumulative disaster exposure and prolonged displacement can affect people (see Box 2-1). Peek likened this process to the effect of experiencing successive concussions, in which the second concussion causes more harm to the human brain than the first concussion. Cumulative trauma is similarly multiplicative—rather than additive—in terms of how it affects a child's life.

A CALL TO ACTION FROM THE NATIONAL COMMISSION ON CHILDREN AND DISASTERS

Peek emphasized that as disasters increase in frequency and magnitude, work to assess the acute and the enduring effects of these events on children's lives has never been more urgent. She described the human suf-

---

BOX 2-1
Effects of Cumulative Disaster Exposure and Prolonged Displacement

- Worsened mental health symptoms
- Higher risk of major physical health problems
- Amplification of the effect of future collective trauma exposures
- Negative behavioral outcomes among adults
- Cumulative vulnerability, or a "declining trajectory," among children

SOURCE: Peek presentation, July 22, 2020.

fering on full display after Hurricane Katrina as activating the collective conscience of the nation. Peek stated that "the emergency response, academic, and policy communities sprang into action to provide life-sustaining resources and generate life-saving knowledge." Peek said that for child and disaster researchers and practitioners, arguably the most important intervention to come out of that disaster was the creation of the presidentially appointed NCCD that developed groundbreaking interim and final reports (Lavin et al., 2009; NCCD and AHRQ, 2010). The final report included a call for a National Strategy on Children and Disasters and recognized the unique needs of children affected by disasters:

> The Commission respectfully calls on the President to develop and present to Congress a National Strategy on Children and Disasters…. The strategy would sound an unequivocal call to action to engage one another around a cohesive set of meaningful national goals and priorities to remedy the years of benign neglect of children. The unique needs of children must be more thoroughly integrated into planning and made a clear and distinct priority in all disaster management activities. (NCCD and AHRQ, 2010)

Citing research conducted by Save the Children and other groups,[1] Peek said that real progress has been achieved on certain fronts in response to the concrete recommendations that were made in the commission's influential report. However, she noted that in the decade since its publication, many of the recommendations have not been acted on. Peek described 2020 as an age of extremes—not only environmental extremes, extreme social and economic inequality, and extreme political and public division, but also a moment of extreme social engagement and action. Some of the largest peaceful protests in U.S. national history have been taking place, with helping behavior and mutual aid being offered across generations and on an unprecedented scale. This historic moment is an opportunity to establish a new NCCD to follow up on the historic contributions of the 2010 report, said Peek. She suggested that this follow up should place children's voices, perspectives, creativity, contributions, and rights in the center of the discussion.

Rationale for Placing Children's Voices in the Center of the Discussion

Peek outlined three reasons why it is urgent that children's voices be placed in the center of research, practice, and policy making in this area. First, children are the experts on their own lives and thus there is much to

---

[1] More information about Save the Children is available at https://www.savethechildren.org (accessed October 23, 2020).

learn from them; in this respect, they are an enormous resource. She and colleagues analyzed news media coverage of children's contributions after Hurricane Katrina and determined that children donated or raised more than $471 million in Katrina relief. Furthermore, children helped generate more than 14,000 toy donations, organized the collection of more than 23,000 books and 400 reading kits, and volunteered time and labor after Katrina. She added that those estimates were limited to those included in media coverage, so it does not encompass countless efforts children made that were not covered by the press. Secondly, Peek argued that children's voices should be more carefully placed in the center of these efforts because, despite their many contributions, children are typically excluded from decision-making activities that will affect them now and well into the future. For instance, children do not vote and are excluded from the very decision-making processes that will have a profound influence on their health, safety, and well-being now and into the future (Anderson, 2005; Peek, 2008). Thirdly, she maintained that if children are not included in this crucial, historic moment, then the opportunity to harness the creativity, courage, compassion, and energetic commitment of one-fourth of the nation's population will be squandered. Peek explained that to forge a path through the multiple cascading crises of today's world, everyone will need to work together—including children and youth populations—across the divisions that typically keep groups apart and prevent them from recognizing their interdependence with one another. She urged participants to continue uplifting the voices and needs of children and youth and acting on their behalf.

DISCUSSION

Lavin noted that NCCD did not speak directly with children during their deliberations. She asked Peek if she recommends that the potential follow-on commission have conversations with children. Peek replied that after Hurricane Katrina and every large-scale disaster since, child- and youth-led groups have mobilized. In fact, after Hurricane Katrina, there were so many child- and youth-led groups in New Orleans that an umbrella organization was created to help organize them. She emphasized that children are organizing and making contributions in many spheres of society. Thus, if there is a presidentially-appointed follow-on commission to NCCD, Peek not only recommended that the adult commissioners speak to children and youth, but that a diverse range of children and youth be made a core part of the commission's work.

Lavin asked whether adolescents make up the majority of youth who volunteer and act in response to disasters. Peek emphasized the importance of taking an intersectional approach to all analyses and noted that in their analysis of 10 years of newspaper coverage of children's contributions in the aftermath of Katrina, her team at the Natural Hazard Center looked at the ages of children involved. They found that contributions were not limited to teenagers, who have more autonomy than younger children. Children as young as preschoolers were engaged in support activities (e.g., by collecting pennies to send penny jars to the Gulf Coast). The analyses showed that children and youth were contributing across the age spectrum, as well as having diversity across race, ethnicity, and gender.

In the context of exploring matrices for evaluating response and recovery efforts related to social and human services, Lavin asked about any ongoing efforts to study groups of children postdisaster to document the development of those most affected. Peek responded that social sciences research around disasters has shown that having the capacity to volunteer and help can promote postdisaster recovery. For example, Steffen and Fothergill (2019) analyzed the effects of volunteerism after the 9/11 terrorist attacks and found that volunteering helped to put people on the recovery trajectory. Other researchers have been documenting disaster-specific case studies of children after disasters such as the Joplin tornado, Hurricane Katrina, and Superstorm Sandy. Peek highlighted the need for cross-scale, cross-geographic, and cross-disaster comparisons to help identify points of commonality and differences among disasters across time and scale.

Heather Beal, founder and president of BLOCKS Inc., noted that the Federal Emergency Management Agency (FEMA) has a Youth Preparedness Council for high school students;[2] she asked Peek about the possibility of establishing a similar council for elementary and middle school students. Lavin asked about research to assess the effect of the Youth Preparedness Council. Peek was unaware of studies that systematically assessed the progress of the youth council participants and leaders over time, but she suggested that researchers should do so. She noted the Blizzard Bag project, organized by the FEMA Region VIII Youth Council leader, was able to reach thousands of children and youth across the state of Colorado to help them prepare for blizzards. That youth leader is now studying engineering in college and has continued his commitment to emergency preparedness planning, she added.

Peek commented that she and her graduate students were prompted to conduct the bottom-up analysis of children's contributions after Hurricane Katrina by their participation in Stefanie Haeffele and Virgil Storr's book, *Bottom-Up Responses to Crisis* (Haeffele and Storr, 2020). In that chapter, Peek and colleagues wrote about how children are creating change from the bottom up. She then co-authored a chapter in *Government Responses*

---

[2] More information about FEMA's Youth Preparedness Council is available at https://www.ready.gov/kids/youth-preparedness-council (accessed October 23, 2020).

to Crisis (Peek and Domingue, 2020) about top-down actions of federal programs focused specifically on children and disasters, which examined whether the focus was on mitigation, preparedness, response, or recovery. Peek highlighted a gap in mitigation programs for children and youth, noting that federal partners tend to focus on emergency preparedness and response. However, she added that FEMA and other federal agencies have child- and youth-focused programs that are bringing more children into the natural hazard space than ever before.

Lavin asked about strategies to build the evidence base for continuity and restoration of social and human services. Peek replied that the first step is to take stock of what is already happening in the field, thereby building important connections and understanding the work of other organizations in order to set an agenda for action. "We cannot change the landscape if we do not understand the current status of the landscape," she said.

3

Effect of Disasters on Critical Child Infrastructure

Children and families have unique needs in disaster response and recovery. The second panel of the workshop aimed to consider how the systems and networks of social and human services that serve children and youth are affected during and after a major federally declared natural or environmental disaster; participants also explored how services are delivered during and after a disaster. The panel was moderated by Robert Amler, dean of the New York Medical College School of Health Sciences and Practices.

OFFICE OF CHILD CARE AND THE CHILD CARE DEVELOPMENT FUND

Shannon Christian, director of the Office of Child Care (OCC) at the Department of Health and Human Services' (HHS's) Administration for Children and Families (ACF), provided an overview of the Child Care Development Fund (CCDF) administered by OCC. She described OCC's role in disaster preparation and response, from requiring disaster plans of grantees to offering grant flexibilities after an event to providing coordination and technical support.

Overview of the Child Care Development Fund

Christian explained that OCC administers the CCDF, which is a $8.7 billion block grant from the federal government to state, territorial, and tribal grantees to help eligible low-income families pay for child care for children from birth through age 12. Grantees must reserve a minimum set of funding to improve the quality of care for all children, which can also be used in responding to disasters. Combined with funds from state matching, maintenance-of-effort funding, and Temporary Assistance for Needy Families (TANF) transfers, the grant totals $11.7 billion. Christian noted that the CCDF provides grantees with flexibilities in program design. Some program areas must be designed within federal parameters, including the population subsets grantees can focus on, as well as provider payment rates, parent copay amounts, and eligibility criteria. Other components of program design are flexible. The CCDF also has a set percentage of funds from Congress that can be used to support the development of research and technical assistance centers, which include staff dedicated to emergency and disaster plan development and support.

Grantee Disaster Plans

CCDF grantees are required to develop disaster plans for preparedness, response, and recovery, said Christian. Plans must include policy and capacity to continue paying child care providers when a child care program is closed because of a disaster. Guidelines for the continuation of child care services must be outlined, which may include the provision of emergency and temporary child care services and temporary operating standards during a disaster and recovery. Response provisions must include how grantees will use the assistance program's flexibility in making changes to their child care assistance program. In addition, plans must outline procedures for evacuation, relocation, shelter in place, and lockdown. Recovery activities include building the supply of child care after a disaster. Christian noted that one method of increasing supply is to provide grants to providers to reopen classrooms and serve additional children. OCC provides technical assistance to grantees to improve these disaster plans.

Office of Child Care Responses to Disasters

OCC provides technical assistance to grantees to help them understand and use flexibilities available in their child care funds, said Christian. OCC also coordinates support for grantees in partnership with ACF and other federal government programs, such as the Federal Emergency Management Agency (FEMA). Additionally, OCC helps grantees identify national organizations that can provide support, such as Save the Children, the American Red Cross (ARC), and Child Care Aware of America. One of OCC's major roles is to coordinate support, while the state, tribe, or territory takes the lead in conducting on-the-ground response activity.

Child Care Development Fund Flexibilities to Address Disasters

Christian outlined certain flexibilities in the use of CCDF funds that come into play during disasters and emergencies. In these events, a state, territory, or tribal grantee can change the eligibility or priority criteria for services. This can be done via income threshold adjustments for subsidy eligibility and exclusion of disaster and temporary assistance from income considerations. Furthermore, parent copays can be waived. Grantees can broaden the definition of protective services to include children affected by a federal or state-declared emergency, thereby waiving eligibility criteria, such as work/training requirements, for child care services.

Christian noted that quality dollars (i.e., the funds grantees are required to set aside to improve child care for all children) can be used to provide immediate child care assistance to displaced families. Flexibility also allows grantees to eliminate the quality spending percentage in order to redirect those funds to direct services. CCDF grants can always be used to fund mental health consultants and trauma training as part of professional development, she added. Grantees can provide supply-building grants to child care providers to be used for equipment, supplies, professional development and staffing, minor repair and remodeling, and ongoing financial assistance while a provider is rebuilding.

Although using most of these flexibilities requires obtaining waivers or plan amendments, this can be done retroactively. Grantees can also request temporary waivers for extraordinary circumstances, which temporarily exempt grantees from meeting specific requirements. Finally, states have the flexibility to use TANF for child care services. Christian noted that this is not under OCC control and that TANF may have fewer requirements than CCDF and therefore may be better suited to emergency use in some cases.[1]

Supplemental Funding

Christian said that in a disaster, OCC can access additional funding. For example, after the federally declared natural disasters in 2018 and 2019, OCC received $30 million in supplemental funding for grantees affected by these events. Grantees received funding by way of an application process, which could include retroactive funds for documented expenses. This was the first time that OCC received direct supplemental disaster funding appropriated specifically for child care. She suggested that this process will likely be more effective than directing monies to partner agencies and hoping they will allocate some of it to child care services. Recently, the

---

[1] More information about flexibilities related to these funding streams is available at https://www.acf.hhs.gov/occ/resource/im-2017-02 (accessed October 29, 2020).

Coronavirus Aid, Relief, and Economic Security (CARES) Act allocated $3.5 billion to OCC to enable grantees to address COVID-19, she added.

Challenges in Supporting Children Affected by Disasters

The COVID-19 pandemic ushered in new challenges that were not part of grantee emergency and disaster plans, said Christian. For example, some states ordered providers to close completely or limit services solely to essential workers, and concerns of virus spread led some centers to opt to close. As of July 2020, many had yet to reopen and many of those that had reopened had far fewer children. Christian stated that funding from the CARES Act is being used to meet new demands on child care systems, including (1) serving children of essential workers; (2) sustaining the child care industry in spite of reduced numbers of children served; (3) making hygiene products such as masks, gloves, hand sanitizer, and cleaning solutions available; and (4) installing safety measures (e.g., space dividers) between napping children.

Challenges also stem from the way the COVID-19 pandemic appears to be changing the nature of child care, said Christian. Although the influence of pandemic-related parent safety concerns on the supply and demand for child care is not yet fully understood, there seems to be an increased preference for small settings, such as child care providers offering services in their homes and smaller child care centers. Furthermore, recommended safety policies and practices are raising costs while decreasing revenue for these providers, Christian added. For example, social distancing results in fewer children per classroom, thereby increasing the cost per child. Other expenses are incurred by sanitation screening, arrival and departure procedures where teachers walk children to and from the classroom to avoid having parents inside the building, and the increased staffing needs associated with hand washing between all activities. She added that because of changes in the child care funding model, both open and closed centers are requesting support in order to remain in business until the economy reopens.

Christian outlined several additional challenges that were faced before the COVID-19 pandemic. Stating that child care is "a market, not a program," she explained that this industry is a varied mix of public and privately funded organizations that are not coordinated by a single entity. Despite increased awareness of brain science and the effect of adverse childhood experiences, allowable spending on child trauma expert services has not translated into use of this resource on the level it should. Another challenge is the lack of a mechanism for OCC to deploy volunteers to disaster sites to meet the demand. Furthermore, OCC is not close enough to disaster sites to be able to intervene directly. She added that the COVID-19 pandemic has caused uncertainty as to how OCC may need to alter its approach to disaster planning, response, and recovery. Potential changes could include modifying state disaster plan requirements and making internal adjustments to address any future widespread health emergency, she suggested.

DISASTER PLANNING AND COLLABORATION TO SUPPORT CHILDREN, YOUTH, AND FAMILIES

Lauralee Koziol, national advisor on children and disasters at FEMA, described the collaborative disaster planning, response, and recovery efforts needed to support children and families. She highlighted three common ways that children, youth, and families need to be supported after disasters (see Box 3-1). She noted that the need for emotional and mental health support appears to have grown over the past couple of years, but in her own experience the number of children requiring these services seems to have decreased in the past 4 years.

Disaster Planning and Preparedness

Koziol remarked that because disasters begin and end locally, strong local plans can reduce the level of need during response and recovery if they include robust plans for continuity of operations, emergency operations, and recovery. A continuity-of-operations plan (COOP) addresses how to resume business immediately after the disaster and how to communicate with staff and clients in the absence of electricity or Internet service. An emergency operations plan addresses how to meet the needs of the organization, staff, and children and youth under care during an emergency. An emergency operations plan should include procedures for

---

BOX 3-1
Support Needs for Disaster-Affected Children, Youth, and Families

1. Address immediate and unmet needs, such as food and commodities (e.g., infant formula, diapers, wipes).
2. Reestablish infrastructure and support services, including schools, child care, and other human and support services that allow parents and guardians to return to work and help the economy recover.
3. Provide emotional and mental health support.

SOURCE: Koziol presentation, July 22, 2020.

evacuation, communication with parents and guardians, and reunification in the event that children and youth are separated from their parents for a few hours or longer. Additionally, the emergency operations plan should include provisions for sheltering for an extended period of time in the event of infrastructure and road damage. Koziol added that plans should consider scenarios such as sheltering children who may need critical medical care while communication lines are down.

Recovery plans should preidentify resources that will enable services to resume quickly after a disaster, said Koziol. These may include alternate facilities that can be used and community stakeholders who can collaborate as partners. Addressing these aspects of recovery during the planning process provides viable options in the event of a disaster. Recovery plans also include housing important documents in areas where they will not be damaged by a disaster, being aware of insurance plan coverage and deductibles, and having an idea of the documentation that will be required during the insurance claims process. She added that having an ongoing relationship with the local emergency manager can be helpful in identifying resources should a disaster occur. An additional component of recovery planning is familiarity with potential sources of support, such as the Small Business Administration, FEMA public assistance, and provisions for private, nonprofit organizations.

Collaboration in Disaster Response

Koziol maintained that collaboration is one of the most important aspects of disaster response. She added that addressing the needs of children and families should be approached as a joint planning and development effort among FEMA, HHS, the Department of Education, nonprofit organizations, and the private sector. Identifying partners, understanding their programs, and seeing how programs intersect is invaluable, she noted. A disaster will often increase the number of stakeholders involved, which warrants flexibility in accommodating the needs of disaster survivors. Having ongoing working relationships already in place can enable organizations to develop trust and respect for one another, as well as creating a greater breadth of perspectives that can be pooled together for the benefit of survivors, she added.

AMERICAN RED CROSS: SUPPORT FOR CHILDREN ACROSS ALL PHASES OF DISASTERS

Trevor Riggen, senior vice president of disaster cycle services at ARC, described preparedness programs delivered by his organization and described the role that youth can play in helping their families during a disaster. He discussed how ARC's partnerships with smaller organizations with expertise tailored to a community's specific needs can support long-term recovery efforts and highlighted the values of cultural competence and self-determination that drive the organization.

American Red Cross Preparedness Programs

Riggen remarked that children can play a role in changing the culture of preparedness in the United States because they often serve as a catalyst for changing the way a crisis is addressed. To that end, ARC offers three children's preparedness programs. The Prepare with Pedro program, delivered in partnership with FEMA, has been successful in reaching younger children in schools, Riggen said. The Pillowcase Project was born out of Hurricane Katrina, when ARC leadership in Louisiana observed college students stuffing belongings into pillowcases while rushing to evacuate. This program involves visits to classrooms to teach youth how to prepare, stay safe, and remain calm during a crisis. The Sound the Alarm program installs smoke alarms in individuals' homes across the country while educating families on how to exit their homes in a crisis. These programs have demonstrated how children and youth can lead their families by example, he noted. For example, a school superintendent reported that 3 weeks after an in-classroom lesson on staying safe in a house fire, one of the students had a fire in his home. The parents told the superintendent that the only reason they were able to get out was because their son stayed calm and told his parents what to do to exit safely. This exemplifies how an entire community can be thought of as a resource, he said, with children representing "perhaps one of our greatest resources" in disaster preparedness and response.

American Red Cross Response Activities

Riggen noted that ARC is associated primarily with providing response activities, playing a leadership role in FEMA Emergency Support Function 6 by providing and coordinating sheltering, community feeding, and distribution of supplies. However, the provision of health and mental health services is a function of ARC that is often overlooked, he noted. Although the tactical work of sheltering people is often the focus, the health and mental health services provided within the shelters can be one of the most powerful elements of support. He recounted video footage of a family escaping the 2018 Camp Fire in Paradise, California, in which a terrified group is seen driving through debris with flames on both sides of the street. The parents struggle to remain calm, the mother praying out loud, while the children cry in the backseat. In the last 10 seconds of the video, the car emerges from the nearly complete darkness of the smoke into blue skies that represent safety. Riggen said that when he watched the video, his immediate response was imagining their next stop, whether it be an ARC shelter or some other safe haven.

Riggen described how children who must evacuate in such circumstances can experience multiple traumas: escaping the hazard, fearing for their lives, and adjusting to a new and unfamiliar environment. Furthermore, these children may not understand what is happening and may think they are now homeless; they may see their parents struggling to gain some control over their circumstances. ARC is working to help their volunteers and workers better understand the trauma caused by these types of experiences so they can support those children more effectively. He emphasized that while much of the work in the disaster response enterprise focuses on matters of scale—such as how to shelter 10,000 or feed 1 million people—ARC is also trying to drive work at the individual level. Understanding a child's context and emotional experiences creates space and flexibility within which to serve. Volunteers and workers can help individual families and children solve their problems in the moment, rather than treating them as one mass group. He added that when 100 people are treated as a group of 100 people, nuances can be overlooked that could substantially change the outcome for a child who has experienced a large disaster.

American Red Cross Programs to Support Long-Term Recovery

Over the course of ARC's history, the scale of the organization's role in long-term recovery efforts has varied depending on the specific disaster. However, Riggen noted that the past 4 years have been a watershed for ARC's approach to field operations, which is reflected in the organization's establishment of a formal program for long-term recovery. ARC is funded entirely by donations from the public, and long-term operations are established as funding allows. This can take the form of rounds of financial assistance for families, as is currently the case for survivors of Hurricanes Harvey, Florence, Irma, and Maria, as well as the California wildfires. In addition, ARC has established large grant programs and, in some cases, as much as one-third of grant funding is provided to other agencies with more expertise than ARC in specific areas (e.g., serving children).

Riggen provided three examples of ARC grant partnerships that support long-term recovery. One is a nearly complete project in which a large investment from ARC—of more than $40 million over 4 years—was used to place solar panels on 125 schools and to create 30–40 community wells with solar backup power that can remain operational even during a category 5 hurricane. In Puerto Rico, the government (not ARC) operates shelters during disasters, and schools are often used as shelters. The aim of this project was to ensure that schools were (1) safe places for families to be sheltered after a disaster and (2) available for children to return to for classes as quickly as possible. The solar panels provide power and keep water safe for all of the families served by these schools. He added that in the 2 years that some project sites have been up and running, schools have been affected by earthquakes and storms yet have been able to continue operating. An ARC grant provided to HOPE worldwide was used to offer 8-week therapeutic performing arts programs for children directly affected by Hurricane Harvey, primarily in vulnerable neighborhoods across Texas. The positive outcomes from this program demonstrate the benefit of ARC's role in shepherding donor funding to organizations such as HOPE worldwide, said Riggen. Another large grant was provided to California CareForce, a group of volunteer medical professionals that provides free medical, dental, and vision care to those in need at temporary clinics in the wildfire-affected areas. Riggen noted that some recipients may not have had care even before the disaster, but other families lost health care after the disaster as a consequence of losing their jobs, businesses, or other sources of funding necessary to pay for care. This type of recovery work can contribute meaningfully to families' long-term recovery, he said.

An Individualized Perspective on Disaster Services

Riggen illustrated the individualized perspective that ARC brings to disaster services by sharing the story of a 10-year-old named Destiny. Displaced by Hurricane Dorian, Destiny and her family were in a shelter in Georgia. Riggen's colleague saw her talking to her parents while peering out from beneath the covers on her cot. He said that her hiding did not stem from a desire to avoid people, but because she had sensory overload. The noise and chaos in shelters and other environments can simply be too much for many children. Destiny was struggling to cope with sensory overload while her parents were focused on the multiple issues faced by their family. Fortunately, the shelter had sensory kits and ARC was able to provide Destiny with a weighted blanket, a stress ball, and headphones to play music and drown out the noise of the shelter. ARC workers saw a complete turnaround in Destiny within a few hours. Riggen commented that this simple intervention exemplifies ARC's individualized approach and reflects the need to design and deliver care in a way that is responsive to individual needs and values. This includes both cultural competence and the cultural humility to provide authority and self-determination to those ARC serves, he added. The focus is not on the number of meals that can be brought into a shelter, but rather on understanding people's condition, which extends beyond their needs to include their skills and experiences. Riggen emphasized that serving people should include giving them some power and authority over their own experiences.

DISASTER MEDICINE INFRASTRUCTURE PLANNING: HEALTH CARE SYSTEM CONSIDERATIONS FOR CHILDREN

Drawing from two decades spent working in disaster medicine and planning, David Markenson, director and medical director of the Center of Excellence in Precision Responses to Bioterrorism and Disasters, New York Medical College, discussed disaster medicine infrastructure planning with a focus on health care system considerations for children. He shared challenges faced by pediatric systems in planning for response, mitigation, and recovery, and he suggested strategies for improvement.

General Pediatric System Challenges

Many of the planning challenges related to pediatrics stem from a "plan for the population and later address special populations" approach, said Markenson. This perspective is problematic because it can lead to unaddressed needs among special populations and it overlooks special populations as part of the population at large. Recent data indicate that at least 26 percent of the U.S. population is children and youth, with more than 20 million Americans under the age of 6 years.[2] Many of these young children are infants, who have their own set of challenges.

Markenson noted that disaster planning and research efforts have traditionally focused on adults, in large part because of the dearth of data on pediatric and other special populations. Much of the relevant research—especially as it pertains to environmental hazards and terrorism—has come from the military; thus, it does not include data on pediatrics. Similarly, pharmaceutical, medical, and population research typically focuses on adults first in considering planning, preparedness, and access. He described an example of the exclusion of pediatric populations from disaster planning. When the Response Federal Interagency Operation Plan was being developed and federal agencies were being assigned roles, only operational entities were given a role in planning.[3] The Department of Education was primarily a grant funding agency to education entities at the time, so it was not part of the planning process and had no primary role. Even when children are included in planning, those with special health care needs are generally excluded and their medical, mental health, and access issues

---

[2] While a source for these exact numbers was unavailable, more information on demographic trends is available on the Kaiser Family Foundation website at https://www.kff.org/other/state-indicator/distribution-by-age/?currentTimeframe=0&selectedRows=%7B%22wrapups%22:%7B%22united-states%22:%7B%7D%7D%7D&sortModel=%7B%22colId%22:%22Location%22,%22sort%22:%22asc%22%7D (accessed December 18, 2020).

[3] More information about the Response Federal Interagency Operation Plan, 2nd ed., is available at fema.gov (accessed December 18, 2020).

are not addressed. This provides context for some of the challenges faced in pediatric response efforts, he added.

Pediatric Health Care System Challenges

Markenson characterized health care challenges as fundamentally related to capability and capacity. Several decades ago, emergency medical services had almost no capability for children and, although this has markedly improved over time, emergency medical services capability can be quickly exhausted in a time of challenge. A hospital may be linked to two or three pediatric specialty transport teams, and if a disaster damages that hospital or renders it inaccessible—as was the case with Hurricane Katrina and the Joplin tornado—then the teams are no longer available. He explained that hospital capability is also a challenge. The advent of children's hospitals has greatly advanced pediatric care, but it has also created a disaster gap. Even as capacity and capability have increased in pediatric hospitals, they have decreased in nonpediatric hospitals. In many settings, a children's hospital is the only such facility in a town, city, or even a region. Therefore, if a hurricane, tornado, wildfire, electrical event, or other disaster takes out a children's hospital, young patients will be sent to nonpediatric hospitals. It is incumbent upon all hospitals to have the capability to handle the needs of children during a disaster, he said.

Capability limitations also apply to specialty care, said Markenson. For instance, in the United States, burn care is limited and can become unavailable during disasters; this is especially true for pediatric burn capability. As a critical care physician, he has struggled to find rehabilitation facilities for children during typical times. When a system is taxed by increased numbers of children in need during a disaster, these services become even more difficult to access. He added that surge capacity is also affected by capability limitations. If a system's capacity is limited during nondisaster times, it will not be able to adequately handle the surge in patients during a disaster. Markenson explained that in some communities, an event that simultaneously injures four or five children would exceed capacity and be considered a mass casualty event, while an event would have to injure hundreds of adults to be considered a mass casualty event and compromise care.

Disaster Planning for Child Congregate Facilities

Markenson highlighted the need for greater consideration of child congregate facilities in disaster planning, given that children spend much of their time at schools and other facilities. Despite recent improvements in planning and providing resources for emergency and COOPs for businesses, parallel processing planning for children and child congregate facilities has not received the same consideration or resourcing. Even when a setting has a good plan in place—which is rare—systems and plans that are disrupted can fail quickly, he warned. Both research and anecdotal experiences during disasters demonstrate that many parents do not know the emergency plan for their child's school and, even if they do, most will disregard official emergency evacuation plans and instead go directly to where their child is. Even when the setting has a plan to take children to a safe place for reunification, many parents go against orders to retrieve their children, which can disrupt child movement. These issues are rooted in lack of communication and can place the plan for an entire community at risk of failure, he added.

Although some schools are improving their plans and systems, many challenges remain. To illustrate, Markenson described a procedure he conducts when he visits emergency management offices. When asked where shelters are likely to be created if there is a need, schools are almost always first, second, or third on the list of potential shelter sites. During separate meetings with school officials, he asks about the school's plan for its students in the event of a natural disaster. Typically, the plan is to evacuate the schools and send children home. Therefore, in the event of a disaster, children would be moved out of their schools to their homes, and then additional resources would be needed to bring family units back from homes to the schools. It is commendable that schools generally have some plans in place, problematic though they may be, he added. Other types of child congregate facilities (e.g., camps, after-school programs, religious settings) are largely without plans or adequate resources.

Ways to Address Pediatric System Challenges

Markenson suggested several ways to address the challenges facing the pediatric health care system. The disaster response system lacks adequate pediatric-specific supplies and resources, such as diapers and formula, which needs to be addressed. Family units are excluded when the planning approach is to focus on "population first" and others second. Instead, disaster planning should consider families as units: families do not want to be separated during routine times, much less during a disaster. Plans should recognize that during the day, most parents will be at work and children will be at congregate facilities; therefore, families will need to be reunited. Additionally, until families are together, they will need to be assured that they will be reunited. Coordination of support for children across all sectors also needs consideration in planning, he added. The local, state, and federal levels should all have pediatric-specific plans, resources, and tools. At the federal level, this includes ensuring appropriate focus and expertise regarding children's issues, as well as equipping the Strategic National Stockpile with necessary pediatric resources and supplies.

DISCUSSION

Changing the Culture to Focus on Supporting Children's Needs

Patricia Frost, National Pediatric Disaster Coalition, asked how the systemic culture of prioritizing adults over children can be appropriately rebalanced in the emergency management, hospital, and first-responder community. Markenson replied that this process begins with how the makeup of the population is conceived. Often, the problem begins with the concept of "the population" being comprised of adult males aged 18–55 years, without recognizing that 25–30 percent of the population is comprised of children and youth. He maintained that any local, state, or federal organization with a legal responsibility to plan should, by definition, direct 30 percent of its effort, time, and resources to children. Changing the culture begins with the obligation to prepare for the population and recognize the percentage of children and youth within the general population, he added.

A participant asked Koziol whether she has seen any changes in the years since Hurricane Katrina in how federal emergency managers work to identify and support the needs of children. Koziol replied that she has seen change evolve slowly over time. For example, FEMA did not focus on children until 2009–2010. At that time, the approach was to build resources throughout programs and then partner with governmental agencies such as HHS or the Department of Education. Progress has been made since then, but there is still work to be done, especially in training and further socialization.

A participant asked if the change in the CCDF requirements that required grantees to develop an emergency plan served to increase awareness of the importance of emergency preparedness and planning among child care providers or lead state agencies for child care. Christian replied that it has, noting that when this requirement was strengthened in the 2014 reauthorization, several states asked to update their disaster plans. Furthermore, ACF now brings more attention to disaster plans by reviewing them as part of the onsite monitoring process, as well as offering trainings at conferences that are generally well attended. She added that the COVID-19 pandemic has increased interest in this area, because planning and response efforts that were adequate for previous events are not sufficient for the pandemic response.

Restoration and Continuity of Child Care

In the context of the importance of restoring and ensuring continuity of child care after a disaster, a participant asked which entity is responsible for assessing child care facilities to ensure that they are safe for the return of children and staff. Christian clarified that depending on the specific issue, the safety of facilities is a state or local responsibility rather than a federal one. She said that child care is necessary for recovery after a disaster. While many natural disasters have a smaller scope than is currently the case with COVID-19, the need for child care is common among affected families. Parents often require child care while they are involved in disaster-related tasks, such as dealing with what is left of their homes, going through the paperwork process, and standing in lines at agencies. Child care is sometimes provided at the disaster site itself, funded by ACF, ARC, and other organizations. However, it is important to restore normal child care services as soon as possible. Christian added that extra support and training are needed to support teachers and children who may be traumatized.

Addressing Challenges Related to Reunification

A participant asked for suggestions to improve communication with parents and guardians about reunification. Markenson replied that the major missing element is communicating the plan to parents. In his experience both as a professional who visits schools and as a parent of children attending elementary, middle, and high schools, he has not seen information shared during orientation or the school year about what would happen during an emergency. A parent's social and behavioral goal is naturally to get to their child immediately in an emergency, so parents will go to whatever location they know their child will be. He added that parents will go directly to a reunification site if they know that the children will be moved to that location and it is the only way to reunite with their child.

Riggen noted that after Hurricane Katrina and other disasters, the focus shifted to the use of technology for reunification. Although technology can be useful, it can also blind people to the simple challenges of staying connected. He suggested that expectations regarding communications should be established prior to a disaster so that they are understood by both parents and children. Parents should be aware of the reunification location and know what the messaging will look like, so they will not question the validity of a text or other communication they receive. He added that technology tools including ARC's Safe and Well website,[4] Facebook, and other social media sites can be helpful; however, the formal plan needs to be well understood by everyone involved prior to a crisis situation. This can be achieved by communicating the plan well ahead of time and on a regular basis throughout the year so that families know what to expect.

---

[4] ARC's Safe and Well website is available at https://safeandwell.communityos.org/cms/index.php (accessed October 23, 2020).

Christian asked if ARC teams are in contact with individual child care providers about the plan for reunifying children with parents after a disaster that occurs during a child care day. Riggen replied that the coordination strategy depends on the setting and other circumstances. ARC partners with agencies that are in communication with many different providers in order to stay connected. He added that most ARC shelters are open for 24–36 hours, but some recent large-scale disasters have required extended sheltering of 2–3 months. In extended sheltering situations, ARC collects information from families to assist them in reaching out to providers to learn their plan for resuming child care services. He added that health services workers often provide this assistance because they are accustomed to handling confidential information and working through channels and processes.

4

Exploring the Gaps in Evidence

Although the body of data and evidence on children and disasters has increased since Hurricane Katrina, many gaps remain. This session of the workshop featured three presentations that explored the gaps in the knowledge base related to the delivery of services to children after disasters. The discussion included specific gaps that persist, emergency function support status, uniform data collection and sharing methods, and school-based clinics. The session was moderated by Heather Beal, founder and president of BLOCKS Inc.

PROGRESS AND GAPS IN SUPPORTING CHILDREN, YOUTH, FAMILIES, AND SERVICE PROVIDERS

Lori Peek, director of the Natural Hazards Center and professor at the University of Colorado Boulder, provided an overview of federal programs addressing child, youth, and family needs; identified gaps in knowledge; and highlighted opportunities to address those gaps. She also described an ongoing project focused on identifying federal resources targeting children and disasters.[1] Such resources have increased since Hurricane Katrina, and

---

[1] Peek noted that much of the information she presented is drawn from a chapter she co-authored called "Recognizing Vulnerability and Capacity: Federal Initiatives Focused on Children and Youth Across the Disaster Life Cycle," which is a summary and descriptive analysis of all federal programs geared specifically for children and youth, as well as available guidance documents aimed at caregivers, child care centers, schools, and other child-centric institutions (Peek and Domingue, 2020).

children are increasingly recognized as both being vulnerable and having the capacity to engage in emergency management activities.

Federal Programs Addressing Child, Youth, and Family Needs

Peek and colleagues conducted an exhaustive Internet search and collaborated with federal government colleagues working on child-centered programs to assess the federal resources available that focus on children and disasters (Peek and Domingue, 2020). For each resource identified, they collected the following information: the name of the program, document, or resource; the sponsoring agency; a program overview; and the target age group of the program or audience. This enabled them to determine whether more resources are targeting younger children or teens and whether the audience is children and youth or adult caregivers. They found that Hurricane Katrina caused a dramatic shift in terms of a focus on children and families, said Peek. Since 2005, numerous federal agencies have offered programs or guidance documents for the benefit of children experiencing disasters,[2] and children are increasingly being recognized as resources as well as a vulnerable group. Instead of characterizing children as victims, efforts are now engaging the capacity of children in emergency management activities. Many agencies offer child- and disaster-focused educational programs and guidance documents aimed at parents, schools, child care centers, and child service providers.

Gaps and Opportunities in Federal Programs for Children and Disasters

Peek also identified gaps and the opportunities in federal programs that focus on children and disasters. Currently, most programs and documents focus on individual or household preparedness and emergency planning and response. Many do not use participatory activities, and there is a tendency to treat children as a monolithic group. Peek outlined opportunities to shift this service landscape. She put forward the idea that participatory programs should be best practice because children and youth learn and retain information most effectively through those types of programs. Thus, there is an opportunity to increase the active engagement of children and youth when developing guidance documents, curricular programs, and other resources.

---

[2] These agencies include the Centers for Disease Control and Prevention, the Department of Education, the Department of Health and Human Services, the Department of Homeland Security, the Department of Justice, the Environmental Protection Agency, the Federal Bureau of Investigation, the Federal Emergency Management Agency, the National Institutes of Health, the National Oceanic and Atmospheric Administration, the National Weather Service, the U.S. Army Corps of Engineers, and the U.S. Geological Survey (Peek and Domingue, 2020).

Additionally, most of the programs focus on personal or household preparedness. Peek suggested shifting toward collective empowerment models and coproduction of services to consider individuals within interconnected webs of families and communities, rather than considering them in isolation. She added that teaching children and youth how entire communities can work together to achieve change can promote preparedness for children, families, schools, and child care centers. Child-serving institutions also warrant greater focus, as much of the available guidance is centered around individual children or households. Another gap is that most of the available programs focus on emergency planning and response, with far less guidance on recovery. Peek contended that children, youth, and those who care for them can engage in mitigating disaster losses and be involved in long-term recovery efforts. Finally, Peek said that children are often depicted as a monolithic group, without taking their full diversity into account. She recommended an intersectional lens be used to consider the incredible diversity within the child population.

Support for Service Providers: Building Capacity Among Voluntary Organizations Active in Disaster

Peek described a project to build capacity among voluntary organizations active in disaster (VOADs) to provide support for service providers and protect children in emergencies. In partnership with Save the Children (STC), the Natural Hazards Center is conducting a collaborative project focusing on VOADs. She explained that the Natural Hazards Center and STC recognize and honor the role VOADs play in delivering services to affected communities, and the aim of the project is to build the capacities of VOADs to ensure that children's needs are considered. Beginning with two initial focal states, the project is currently being carried out in Nebraska and Arkansas. Project goals include (1) assessing child-specific knowledge, skills, and attitudes in two state VOADs; (2) increasing the knowledge and awareness of children's needs in disasters within VOADs and emergency management; (3) advancing the prioritization of children's needs and abilities to meet those needs in VOADs and emergency management organizations; and (4) assessing project interventions.

Peek said that according to initial surveys they conducted, VOADs reported relatively low levels of knowledge about children and youth in disaster and had relatively small skill sets in working with this population, yet they had high levels of desire to learn more about children and youth. STC is leading project efforts to increase VOAD and emergency management knowledge and awareness of children's needs in disasters by developing and implementing interventions that are then assessed by the Natural Hazards Center to determine whether project goals are achieved.

Assessment involves baseline surveys, participatory asset mapping with VOAD members, and geographic information system mapping using the Centers for Disease Control and Prevention (CDC) social vulnerability index to determine where potentially vulnerable children are located within each state. Additionally, the Natural Hazards Center is performing social network analysis (SNA) to understand how VOADs are enhancing and deepening communication, cooperation, coordination, and collaboration. The Natural Hazards Center is also examining how much engagement exists between nonmember, child-serving organizations and VOAD member organizations, as well as looking at the child-specific resource exchanges between VOAD member organizations and child-focused experts in comparison to VOAD member organizations' other resource exchanges.

SNA categorizes resources into four groups: information, equipment, training, and child-specific resources, said Peek. Analysis indicated that of these categories, VOADs reported that they seek information from one another most frequently and that they seek child-specific resources the least frequently, with some VOADs seeking no child-specific resources. Peek hypothesized that these organizations are not seeking child-specific resources because they are not accessible, rather than a perceived lack of need for them. When VOADs do seek child-specific resources, SNA data revealed that they all seek it from the same node—STC. Peek suggested that if there were more well-integrated child–expert nodes, then child-specific information-seeking activity would increase commensurately. She emphasized that these types of expansive gaps can be bridged by bringing resources and expertise together.

STUDY OF THE EFFECT OF HURRICANE MARIA ON CHILDREN IN PUERTO RICO

Amanda Rivera, executive director of the Youth Development Institute of Puerto Rico (YDI) (see Box 4-1), described her organization's efforts to assess the impact of disasters on families, especially those living in poverty, that can be exacerbated by disaster. She outlined the effects of Hurricane Maria on food security, early care and education, and the coordination of services among stakeholders, and she highlighted opportunities to address service gaps during future disasters. She explained that YDI, a partner of the KIDS COUNT project, is both an advocacy entity and a think tank; this hybrid organization was formed because of the lack of entities carrying out policy, research, and advocacy work in Puerto Rico.

Rivera said that when Hurricane Maria hit Puerto Rico, YDI was aware of the disproportionate impact that this massive event would have on children living in poverty. In response to the disaster, two initiatives were developed: A study on the effect of Hurricane Maria on children, and

> **BOX 4-1**
> **Youth Development Institute of Puerto Rico**
>
> The Youth Development Institute of Puerto Rico (YDI) is the island's only entity exclusively dedicated to promoting research and public policies that strengthen the economic security of families with children and youth. YDI's goal is to drastically reduce child poverty on the island and ensure that all children have opportunities that allow them to live in homes with economic security. This organization works to reduce child poverty by empowering those affected to engage in the policy process, promoting the use of data among policy makers, and activating traditional advocacy work and grassroots mobilization to raise awareness of the problem and its solutions.
>
> SOURCE: http://juventudpr.org/index.html (accessed October 30, 2020).

the Puerto Rico Children and Youth Task Force. The comprehensive study conducted a representative qualitative survey to understand the areas most affected. The children and youth task force began via a joint effort of the Administration for Children and Families (ACF) and STC. The two initiatives revealed three major effects of Hurricane Maria: reduced food security, reduced child care, and reduced coordination of services. This task force continues to operate and is engaged in the Columbia University Resilient Children/Resilient Communities project to conduct preparedness work at the central, island-wide level. They are beginning work on economic security as well as COVID-19 response activities, she added.

Demographic Context of Children in Puerto Rico During Hurricane Maria

Families with children living in poverty are the most affected by disasters caused by natural phenomena, said Rivera. When Hurricane Maria occurred, 58 percent (343,000) of Puerto Rico's children were living in poverty.[3] Rivera pointed out this rate has only varied by 1–2 percentage points over the past 20–30 years, although demographics can vary by jurisdiction within Puerto Rico. The study confirmed that response and recovery scenarios are more complicated for children living in communities with few resources where the majority of families are living in poverty. Rivera likened this to the effect of demographics on communities in New Orleans

---

[3] More information on the demographic context of children in Puerto Rico is available at YDI | Child Poverty Infographics. See juventudpr.org (accessed April 6, 2021).

after Hurricane Katrina. Of the children living in poverty, 78 percent were in single-parent families, typically headed by a mother. Rivera said that this is relevant in considering the resources and supports that a family has at home. Similarly, of families with incomes up to 130 percent of the poverty level, 29 percent do not qualify for the nutrition assistance program. Furthermore, around 26 percent of low-income children do not have Internet access. Rivera noted that lack of Internet access has become far more pertinent during the current school closings brought on by COVID-19 than it was after Hurricane Maria. When the alternative to a disruption in school is distance learning, Internet access becomes a critical resource. She added that 10 percent of children living in poverty in Puerto Rico have a physical or mental disability or live with a parent who has a disability, which becomes an added vulnerability during a disaster.

Effect of Hurricane Maria on Food Security

Whether it is a hurricane, earthquake, or a pandemic, disasters pose many challenges to food security, said Rivera. Hurricane Maria caused a massive dislocation of the food supply chain that affected people across income levels. The survey revealed that 27.9 percent of people with annual income of $40,000 or less experienced difficulty accessing food after Hurricane Maria; this percentage increased to 38.2 percent among those earning $15,000–$39,999 per year and rose to 50 percent for people earning less than $15,000 per year. Rivera noted that low-income families experience the economic impact of a disaster longer than those in higher income brackets, with many still experiencing food insecurity issues 1 year after the hurricane. When high rates of poverty already affect food security before a disaster, a hurricane will only exacerbate these deficits, she said.

The COVID-19 pandemic has led to school closures in Puerto Rico that have resulted in not only a loss of education, but also a major disruption to food security for families with children. Rivera explained that not all low-income families with children can access nutrition assistance program benefits, but they are able to have meals provided at school. Therefore, school closures and lack of access to lunches for children puts additional strain and pressure on families. She noted that Hurricane Maria also resulted in school closures. The task force found that after the hurricane, benefits from the Special Supplemental Nutrition Program for Women, Infants, and Children (WIC) were being provided via check to most families in Puerto Rico. Because the disaster affected mail delivery, many families faced disruption in accessing those benefits. She added that the lack of electronic benefit transfer (EBT) cards continues to be a challenge today. Additionally, some low-income working families who were already at the brink of poverty before COVID-19 are now facing unemployment and consequent food insecurity.

Opportunities to Ensure Food Security

With these challenges come opportunities to ensure food security after a disaster, Rivera said. For instance, preparedness planning can be conducted in collaboration with volunteer and community-based entities, community leaders, and municipalities. The survey indicated that community-based entities and municipalities were the first line of response supporting families with children. The response from the central government of Puerto Rico came later, followed by the U.S. federal response. She suggested investing in resources and ensuring collaboration among stakeholders to create strong preparedness plans that take into account both food security and the possibility of lengthy disruptions to the food supply chain, as had occurred during Hurricane Maria.

Rivera also advocated for preparedness benefits transfers at the congressional level because many families are living paycheck to paycheck and do not have sufficient income to stock up on supplies and food to prepare for a disaster. Although Puerto Rico does have a policy of advancing benefits before a predicted hurricane, these funds are not sufficient to adequately supply the resources needed for a disaster. Rather than issuing the standard benefit ahead of schedule, she suggested issuing additional benefits to low-income families before an imminent disaster—for example, through the Supplemental Nutrition Assistance Program (SNAP), Temporary Assistance for Needy Families, or WIC. Rivera highlighted a promising development emerging in the EBT infrastructure. In response to the COVID-19 pandemic, EBT cards are being used for families who do not qualify for SNAP but who qualify for free school lunches. Current investment in the EBT infrastructure should be used for emergency transfer, she suggested.

Effect of Hurricane Maria on Early Care and Education

Rivera emphasized that the importance of early care and education is two-fold: it provides children with instructional time and affords parents the economic development opportunity of returning to work. The sooner parents can resume work, the less income they will lose, resulting in greater stability for their families. After Hurricane Maria, the survey collected information on education disruption for children aged 0–5 years. The survey indicated that in Puerto Rico, the majority of child care (70 percent) takes place in informal settings in which the child is cared for by a family member or other adult caregiver. The remaining 30 percent attended Head Start centers (14 percent), public school (8 percent), private school (4 percent), or private or nonprofit child care (2 percent). The average number of disrupted days for children in formal preschool or child care settings after Hurricane Maria was 92 days. Rivera noted that this was greater than the number of days that schools for older children were closed. Furthermore, of the 9.2 percent of children who were receiving early intervention services prior to Hurricane Maria, 70 percent experienced a service interruption and 20 percent have yet to have their early intervention services resume.

A number of factors contributed to the lengthy closures of child care and preschool settings, said Rivera. Many providers lacked basic infrastructure requirements for electricity and water (e.g., backup generators, cisterns) and many parents were unable to pay for the services after the hurricane. Furthermore, the vouchers that some child care centers receive from the government saw a delay in disbursement. Rivera stated that many providers were having cash flow issues before Hurricane Maria and were unable to pay teachers and utilities after the disaster, leading to closures.

Other centers opened with providers working for free as a service to their communities' children and families. Rivera noted that most of the centers are woman-owned small businesses with owners who did an admirable job of continuing to provide services; however, they should not have to work for free. Although the federal government provides many supports, including Small Business Association loans, many people require technical assistance in applying for these supports. She suggested providing additional technical assistance to child care providers around disaster preparedness and recovery. Additionally, for-profit child care centers do not qualify for many of the donations and supports such as power generators and water filtration systems that are made available to nonprofit organizations. Rivera described for-profit child care providers as being in a "gray area" of offering a social service but also operating as a business.

Opportunities to Ensure Continuity of Early Care and Education

Rivera outlined opportunities to ensure continuity of child care centers after a disaster. First, technical assistance and resources for centers should establish robust and feasible continuity-of-operations plans (COOPs). The task force has worked with the Columbia University Resilient Children/Resilient Communities initiative to offer a number of workshops in Puerto Rico on improving COOPs. However, Rivera suggested that the civil sector should not be exclusively responsible for training and education around the development of those plans. She also suggested that emergency grants be disbursed to centers prior to the disaster. This would enable them to prepare and to have cash on hand to withstand the emergency, which may involve months of disruption. She added that small businesses should be provided with assistance in accessing loans and grants for backup generators, solar options, and other equipment that would enable them to become operational more quickly after a disaster.

Effect of Hurricane Maria on Coordination of Services

Rivera explained that the Children and Youth Task Force began with ACF and STC, who then brought nonprofit entities to the table. After Hurricane Maria, ACF and STC organized a series of debriefing meetings in which agencies discussed their efforts and what they were observing. This revealed duplicative efforts and major service gaps, with no way to track populations served. For example, many agencies that focus on housing, family and children services, and education were serving the same population—sometimes targeting the same community. Some communities received resources from agencies multiple times; other communities, particularly those in more remote regions, did not receive any support. When a culture of cross-agency collaboration and coordination is lacking before a disaster, it will be challenging to establish during an emergency, Rivera maintained. Additionally, disaster can lead to a breakdown of all forms of communication, which further complicates these dynamics.

Creating Children and Youth Task Forces to Improve Coordination

Rivera suggested that nonprofit groups be integrated into task forces focused on children and youth to reduce the risk of interagency groups becoming echo chambers, with each agency stating the accomplishments of their organizations. Instead, nonprofit entities should draw attention to communities that are not being served. She outlined several opportunities that can be created by developing task forces:

- Task forces bring government and nonprofit stakeholders together in a consistent, in-person forum to calibrate and coordinate services.
- Task forces can bring community-based entities, service providers, day care centers, nonprofit organizations, and advocates to the table with the government to allow for respectful challenging and dialogue about gaps, both immediately after a disaster and beyond.
- Task forces can facilitate rapid collection of information and identification of gaps.
- A task force can serve as a platform to continue collaboration beyond the disaster, helping partners stay connected.

Rivera also noted several challenges task forces can face. These include ensuring buy-in from government agencies when the task force is outside of the government, balancing both central and regional efforts, and operating without sufficient resources for staffing and supporting participating entities. Additionally, it can be difficult to keep task force members engaged

RESEARCH GAPS IN CHILDREN'S DISASTER MENTAL AND BEHAVIORAL HEALTH

David Schonfeld, developmental–behavioral pediatrician and professor at the University of Southern California and Children's Hospital Los Angeles, examined gaps in children's mental and behavioral health services that persist a decade after recommendations made by the National Commission on Children and Disasters (NCCD). To frame his discussion, he highlighted a recommendation from NCCD's 2010 report:

> The Department of Health and Human Services should enhance the research agenda for children's disaster mental and behavioral health, including psychological first aid, cognitive-behavioral interventions, social support interventions, bereavement counseling and support, and programs intended to enhance children's resilience in the aftermath of a disaster. (NCCD and AHRQ, 2010)

Under this recommendation, NCCD specifically called on the Department of Health and Human Services (HHS) to convene a working group of children's disaster mental health and pediatric experts to review the research portfolios of relevant agencies, identify gaps in knowledge, and recommend a national research agenda across this full spectrum of disaster mental health for children and families. A virtual conference was convened for this purpose, and an informal review of National Institutes of Health grants over the prior 15 years was conducted prior to the conference. This review documented a paucity of funded research on interventions to promote coping and adjustment for children after disasters, he said.

Gaps in Research on the Effects of Disasters on Children's Mental and Behavioral Health

Schonfeld underscored three prominent research gaps pertaining to the effects of disasters on children's mental and behavioral health: (1) research beyond the prevalence of trauma and other mental health symptoms to include a full spectrum of outcomes; (2) efficacy of prevention initiatives involving children and disasters; and (3) intervention for caregivers of children after disaster. Schonfeld and colleagues summarized these findings in a 2018 report (Grolnick et al., 2018).

Effectiveness of Interventions to Promote Behavioral Health and Coping After a Disaster

Schonfeld said that some progress has been made in understanding the effects of disaster on children, but far less is known about the effectiveness of interventions to promote behavioral health and coping after a disaster. Furthermore, the limited intervention studies that were conducted tended to focus on the treatment or prevention of mental illness, especially trauma disorders. Studies on the effects of interventions on distress and bereavement and on the promotion of adjustment, coping, and resilience were critically lacking, he emphasized. Barriers to studying these interventions include the absence of valid measures of outcomes and lack of demonstration of usefulness to research funders and policy makers, he contended. Thus, evidence-based interventions have tended to focus on the prevention or treatment of posttraumatic stress disorder, for which there are validated measures. Schonfeld stated that the report concluded that developing evidence-based interventions for children experiencing disaster is a national priority, and as such, research should be broadened beyond studying the prevalence of trauma, other mental health symptoms, and the effect of trauma approaches. He suggested that the scope of research should expand to include the full spectrum of outcomes (e.g., bereavement, distress that does not reach clinical levels of a mental health diagnosis, adjustment, coping, resilience) as well as the study of interventions in each of these domains. This gap and the urgency to address it persist today, he added.

To highlight this gap, Schonfeld juxtaposed the treatment of trauma and grief responses. Drawing on his visits to New Orleans after Hurricane Katrina and to Paradise, California, after the wildfires and other disasters in the years between, he noted that trauma and grief can co-occur in the lives of children, but he has not seen this overlap mirrored in an overlap in the fields of trauma treatment and childhood bereavement. He contended that grief and trauma are viewed differently. For example, common reactions after the death of a close friend or family member are typically viewed in the mental health field as normative reactions. He explained that while people who are grieving may benefit from support, they are generally considered as not requiring treatment because bereavement is not considered a mental illness. Thus, bereavement support is generally provided by laypeople or faith-based organizations—often at no cost to families—but these professionals generally do not receive reimbursement for the support services they provide. Schonfeld remarked that this type of support is infrequently evaluated through formal research. In contrast, reactions to grief and trauma are often similar, such as experiencing sleep problems and feeling anxious. But when these reactions arise after a person has experienced a traumatic event, they are often viewed as symptoms. When they present in sufficient number and duration, these reactions are then characterized as mental illness such as posttraumatic stress disorder and are seen as requiring treatment. This trauma treatment is provided by licensed and credentialed mental health professionals and is generally covered by health insurance, he said.

While many people accept these distinctions between grief and trauma, a common view voiced by those who have actually experienced traumatic events not involving loss of life is relief that "at least no one died," said Schonfeld. Therefore, suggesting that bereavement is categorically less of a hardship than trauma is inconsistent with the lived experiences of many—if not most—people who have experienced trauma. Furthermore, while adverse childhood experiences as classically construed include parental divorce and incarceration, they do not include the death of a parent. This classification suggests, at some level, that it would be easier to have a parent die than become divorced, even though that is not a commonly held belief. Schonfeld noted that the present workshop has included repeated mention of trauma but far less about the negative effects of loss and other adjustment difficulties.

The National Center for School Crisis and Bereavement and the New York Life Foundation are founding members of the Coalition to Support Grieving Students.[4,5,6] This coalition has 100 organizational members, including top educational and health professional organizations such as the American Academy of Pediatrics and STC. The common conviction of groups in this coalition is that no child should grieve alone, said Schonfeld. To address the need for support, the coalition has developed a wide range of free and publicly available materials, including video-based and print materials for professional development as well as parent and family education.

Efficacy of Prevention Initiatives Involving Children in Disasters

Schonfeld remarked that in the aftermath of disaster, children's stories, coloring books, and parent guides are often developed rapidly and disseminated widely by federal agencies and nongovernmental organizations. However, there is little research on the efficacy of prevention initiatives involving children (Grolnick et al., 2018). He contended that there is generally no preexisting evidence base before initiatives are rolled out nor any attempt to collect evidence to guide future use. This lack of research extends

---

[4] More information about the National Centers for School Crisis and Bereavement is available at https://www.schoolcrisiscenter.org (accessed October 27, 2020).

[5] More information about the New York Life Foundation is available at https://www.newyorklife.com/foundation (accessed October 27, 2020).

[6] More information about the Coalition to Support Grieving Students is available at https://grievingstudents.org (accessed October 27, 2020).

to formal prevention initiatives that educate children on how to prepare for disasters, which are typically promoted for broad use in schools prior to any evaluation.

Schonfeld acknowledged that some students and school personnel may feel empowered and better prepared for possible events after participating in these initiatives. However, children's responses can vary depending on personality, coping style, personal history, and individual vulnerabilities. He explained that while a child receiving training on how to respond in the event of a disaster may feel comforted, this training only provides children with an illusion of control. Furthermore, these efforts could result in increased guilt for the child if they are unable to respond in the idealized fashion in a real event in which a death or serious injury occurs. Thus, Schonfeld advised that these and other unintended consequences be carefully considered and that programs be evaluated more consistently for efficacy before being implemented widely.

Interventions for Caregivers of Children After Disaster

The third research gap identified by Schonfeld and colleagues is the need for more study and intervention for caregivers of children after disaster (Grolnick et al., 2018). He gave the example of a man who shared his story during a training for foster parents in the aftermath of Superstorm Sandy. In response to a discussion about the long-term effects of disasters, this foster father said that he was happily married with a successful career in finance when his toddler became ill and died suddenly. The man said losing his son led him to question many of his life decisions, including his choice of career. Schonfeld noted he is not criticizing the field of finance in repeating this man's realization that while he was making a lot of money, he did not feel he was contributing to society in a way he felt was meaningful. In spite of the high income his job afforded him, he quit and went back to college to become a kindergarten teacher. He found this job, involving shaping the lives of young children, to be extremely rewarding. The man went on to become a foster parent, and he was in the process of adopting a young child when Superstorm Sandy occurred. Schonfeld said this story is not unique, as many individuals that enter child-centered fields such as education, social services, child mental health, pediatrics, and so forth do so in response to experiencing childhood trauma, loss, or some other form of adversity in their own past. In coping with those experiences, they either benefited from the help of others, and want to similarly help someone else, or they recognized the effect that a lack of such assistance had on their own lives and they want to provide another with what they themselves did not receive.

Because this type of service often focuses on ensuring that children receive critical support, Schonfeld hypothesized that a majority of foster and adoptive parents served by ACF and professionals in this field likely have personally experienced trauma and loss. Thus, when disasters occur, prior trauma and loss in the lives of "helpers" in these professions tends to be uncovered. Noting the inherent irony, Schonfeld said that the people who devote their lives to helping children are often those most likely to be hurt personally by doing so. Therefore, he finds the striking lack of evidence-based professional self-care interventions to be a particularly critical gap, especially in professions serving children. He said that a major disaster is not a prerequisite for children to be helped; it can happen on a daily basis. Professionals themselves can be hurt by helping children during a disaster, so professional training and support becomes particularly important, he added.

DISCUSSION

Consequential Research Gaps Since Hurricane Katrina

Beal asked the panel to consider documents such as NCCD's report and events such as Superstorm Sandy, the Paradise wildfires, and Hurricanes Harvey, Irma, and Maria. In reflecting on these documents and events, she asked the panelists what they consider to be the most consequential gap that has been addressed since Hurricane Katrina. Furthermore, she queried what gap they deem to be most important that has yet to close in this same time period.

Schonfeld replied that an important gap that has been addressed is recognition that children are affected by disasters. He contended that before Hurricane Katrina, the effect of such events on children was not given much consideration. Children were viewed as resilient, able to "get over" the disaster, and as not having any significant problems. Schonfeld said this has since been recognized to not be the case. This is evident in the Federal Emergency Management Agency (FEMA) and ACF offering case management and other services around children's needs, as well as in FEMA's creation of a children's coordinator. As discussed in the NCCD report, these steps represent a major advance, said Schonfeld.

In terms of gaps that remain, Schonfeld commented that because it is now understood that adverse experiences cause adversity, more progress is needed on determining how to prevent, support, or ameliorate that adversity. The medical model—involving screening, diagnosis, referral, and treatment for mental illness—has been predominant in interventions. However, research suggests that the vast majority of children who experience disasters are affected. For example, Schonfeld cited research conducted in New York City schools after the 9/11 terrorist attacks, which showed that approximately 87 percent of children had a persistent adjustment problem 6 months after

9/11. Furthermore, of the children who self-identified behavioral health problems and changes in daily functioning, a majority did not seek or receive mental health support within or outside of school. Schonfeld pointed out that these trends occurred despite recovery funding that provided a therapist offering free mental health services in every New York City school. He added that in the current situation of the COVID-19 pandemic, he believes that more than 87 percent of children will be affected and that funding to increase mental health services will not be available. In fact, he surmised that highly constrained budgets will lead to a reduction in mental health staff in order to meet budget shortfalls. Schonfeld concluded that while awareness is good, delivery of supportive services is not following awareness at this point.

Rivera commented that issues of economic insecurity and the effects of poverty on children are still missing from the conversation about disasters. Poverty typically deepens during a disaster in many households with children. Conversations are taking place about trauma and about access to education, but there is a gap in awareness about the effects of poverty on households and children, which are exacerbated by disasters. In thinking about recovery, Rivera maintained that ensuring the economic stability of families must be a priority.

Peek agreed with Schonfeld that progress has been made in increasing awareness of children's needs. She said this workshop, dedicated to children's disaster-related needs, attests to that, as does the progress made in terms of research, service provision, and policy making, much of which traces back to the NCCD report. Peek said that *Children of Katrina*, the book she co-authored with Alice Fothergill of the Department of Sociology at The University of Vermont, describes that children were long depicted in contradictory ways (Fothergill and Peek, 2015). They were either considered as rubber balls, hyper-resilient beings that could bounce back after disaster, or vulnerable victims that had to be completely prepared for and protected. Peek said that NCCD ushered in a much more complex depiction of children and the many systems that surround their lives. She emphasized that this is a major contribution that should not be understated. She added that ensuring educational continuity in the aftermath of disaster—such as categorizing schools as critical infrastructure—is currently the largest gap. She suggested that designating early and childhood education as critical infrastructure would ensure that (1) school buildings are made safe, (2) learning is recognized as a child's primary job, and (3) schools and child care centers would become focal points.

Building Awareness and Action Around Children and Youth in Disasters

Michael Prasad, Barton Dunant Emergency Management Consulting & Training, highlighted the need to build awareness and action around children and disasters among federal, state, county, parish, tribal, and territorial emergency managers. He asked whether children's needs should be considered within the scope of FEMA Emergency Support Functions (ESFs). Peek responded that issues of ESF recognition and integration across ESFs are important to discuss, because the 25 percent of the U.S. population comprised of children stands to benefit.

Schonfeld said that in the work carried out by NCCD, an issue that arose was the prioritization of children's needs. For example, the Strategic National Stockpile was discussed, as well as the major gaps that exist in supplies for children that are attributable to funding shortfalls, among other reasons. Some discussion on stockpile policy focused on having materials that will save the most lives and on making determinations based on "the dollar spent on a life saved," he continued. Children's supplies were often more expensive. For instance, children's medications in liquid format expired more quickly than other forms and were more expensive to store.

Schonfeld referred to a national survey that was conducted to look at general community preferences; it included a question about whether participants would support preparation for a child's needs if that involved a higher cost than preparing for adult needs. The survey respondents demonstrated support for preparing for children's needs. Many people believe that women and children should come first in a disaster, yet federal policy is not following that, he added, noting that parents will risk their lives to try and save their children. Therefore, value placed on children by the general public should be more prominently recognized in disaster preparedness and response planning, Schonfeld contended. Children's needs should be attended to because if children are not taken care of, parents will not take care of themselves. In that sense, responding to children's needs means that adults' needs are simultaneously being met.

This is evident in the current COVID-19 pandemic, he added. Parents want schools to open so that their children are supervised and the parents can return to work, yet they are also worried about their children's safety and want to make sure their children will be taken care of, so they are placing their children's needs first. Lastly, he noted the argument that the needs of children cannot be a focus because children are a special population. Schonfeld maintained that children are not a special population; children are everyone. Childhood is simply a time period in all lives—an important, vulnerable, and critical time period that warrants special attention, he concluded.

Promoting Requirements for Uniform Data Collection

Patricia Frost, National Pediatric Disaster Coalition, asked about how to promote requirements for the adoption of uniform data collection, based on appropriate age groups, that can be used to inform and drive interventions in a disaster. Peek replied that certain organizations or agencies may have specific requirements already, but she is working to promote grassroots, bottom-up data sharing in the academic community. The Natural Hazards Center is encouraging (but not requiring) researchers to publish their data through DesignSafe-CI funded by the National Science Foundation.[7] This platform was predominantly created for engineers, but the Natural Hazards Center has partnered with DesignSafe-CI to ensure it is also accessible to social and behavioral scientists.

Peek said that when data, data collection instruments, and protocols are shared, it expands the potential for comparison across disasters and allows trends and patterns across time and place to be identified. Publisher data events are being organized to encourage social and behavioral scientists to share data when possible, which can be done safely and securely, she added. Rivera said that requirements on *how* data is collected may also help to increase the *amount* of data collected. Many government programs are administered by for-profit and nonprofit service providers that are the recipients of government contracts and grants. When the government is giving providers money to execute a program, requirements to collect data can be attached to grant renewals, she suggested.

Ensuring Adequate Supplies for Children in Shelters

Schonfeld added that when NCCD examined gaps in data collection, it found that FEMA was not routinely inquiring and documenting whether a displaced family had children. Furthermore, shelters did not necessarily have equipment and supplies for children. Even when children's supplies were on hand, the definition of the term *child* tended to include any person aged 0–18 years. Schonfeld noted the food, bedding, and equipment needs are much different for an infant than for a 17-year-old. He recalled an example from his visit to China after an earthquake in Sichuan province that killed 69,000 people in 1 day. There was a photo shared of a female first responder breastfeeding an infant in the rubble. The infant was not her child, but the mother had died and there was no formula, so she breastfed the infant to save their life. While shelters in the United States are likely better equipped, they are not required to be, noted Schonfeld. For instance, a shelter that does not have a supply of infant formula may receive funding for offering sheltering services. Schonfeld suggested that reimbursement to shelters could be tied to meeting minimal requirements in terms of available supplies. Regardless of whether providers are encouraged or required to

---

[7] More information about DesignSafe-CI is available at https://www.designsafe-ci.org (accessed April 6, 2021).

meet the basic needs of children, Schonfeld emphasized that these lifesaving measures must be in place.

Mental Health Support for Children and Youth in Disaster Response and Recovery

Beal asked how active the Puerto Rico Emergency Management Agency was in addressing the gaps Rivera identified. Rivera said that while the agency initially participated in the task force, its engagement lasted only for the first few weeks. She noted that while FEMA was engaged, the local agency was not. She said that for the first 2 months or so after Hurricane Maria, the task force was focused on emergency response, then it swiftly moved to recovery and mental health. Rivera stated that this type of work is not typically considered to be emergency services, but she believes that it should be. She pointed out that after the task force conducted the survey and presented recommendations, the local emergency management agency was receptive.

Donna Wolf, a psychology instructor and school counselor, suggested using school-based mental health centers in high schools to employ youth and "adult anchors" in mitigation and recovery. Schonfeld noted that in addition to school-based mental health centers, there are also school-based clinics that integrate behavioral health services. Professionals such as school nurses examine both psychological and physical issues, which often co-present. Individuals in crisis situations will often have physical symptoms (e.g., stress hormones can cause physical problems like increases in blood pressure, worsening asthma, or a decline in diabetes control). Psychological factors can also present as physical symptoms; typically, an individual in crisis will have some combination of both psychological and physical issues. Schonfeld suggested that both school-based mental health clinics and school-based clinics that integrate mental health providers are mechanisms that can be used effectively. Ideally, students would be able to access an integrated and balanced set of physical health and mental health services. For example, a wellness center was created at Marjory Stoneman Douglas High School after the shooting that occurred there, with mental health providers and one full-time nurse placed in the clinic to offer integrated assessments and services.

Noting the difficulty that families can have in accessing services outside of school, Schonfeld suggested that school-based clinics are often one of the best ways to provide services. However, he pointed out that some families and students prefer accessing services outside of school in order to maintain privacy and have some distance between their school setting and mental health services. Thus, both types of services should be offered in and outside of school as the baseline practice outside of a disaster, Schonfeld said.

Rivera agreed that community mental health support is a major gap, and it would be helpful to provide those services in schools, which are central to communities. An additional concern is the possibility of another major hurricane occurring during the COVID-19 pandemic, during which people are advised not to congregate. The co-occurrence of a hurricane with a pandemic would further complicate mental health challenges experienced by families and simultaneously complicate access to services and community-based support, she added. Schonfeld noted that there have been guidelines developed about sheltering during a natural disaster, such as a hurricane, in the midst of a pandemic. He surmised that they predominantly deal with physical distancing and infection control and less so with the behavioral health aspect of co-occurring disasters. He added that professionals have begun considering how to establish safe shelters during a pandemic because disasters not only co-occur in people's lives, but co-occur in communities.

Peek remarked that the broader question around the efficacy of school-based services is how the resources that children need can be effectively delivered to them. Schools are an obvious mechanism to turn to, but they are already overtaxed in a variety of ways. Additionally, children only spend a certain proportion of their lives in schools. She suggested that considering the issue of where to offer services for children is a prime opportunity to place children's voices and their requests for preferred service locations in the center of the discussion. Questions for children could include "Where are you getting the things you need? Where are the spaces where you feel safe? Who are the advocates and anchors in your life? Who do you trust to provide the things you need?" Peek said that this is an opportunity to learn from children and youth and observe where they are receiving services in order to get vital resources to more of them.

Schonfeld added that individuals who do not have legal status in the United States have particular difficulty accessing services. Many such individuals will not go anywhere that they see as government or government affiliated, including shelters and American Red Cross sites. Thus, the only site that many undocumented people will turn to is their schools. Schonfeld said that several weeks after one of the wildfires, he was meeting with a principal of an affected elementary school. The school had yet to reopen, but she was unpacking water from the trunk of her car, saying that families would only come to the school for safe drinking water. While he commended her for providing this service, he also acknowledged that she was trying to get the school cleaned and reopened while contending with student deaths. Schonfeld said that school leaders cannot be expected to unpack water every morning. Better partnerships must be formed if children and families want to get services at school so that school budgets, resources, and staff are not being used to provide disaster services. He added that after the 9/11 terrorist attacks, he worked with recovery efforts for New York City schools. Some students did not want the school to know that a parent had died on 9/11 because they did not want to be a "9/11 kid." Not all students and staff are comfortable receiving services in schools and people sometimes prefer to access services in a neighboring community where they feel they have more privacy. He agreed with Peek that children and adults need to be able to voice where they want to receive support, and professionals need to provide a menu of options. However, delivering such services requires finances and resources that schools should not be expected to cover when they are already struggling financially, he said.

5

Case Studies: Effect of Disasters on Specific Populations

Workshop participants broke into four groups to discuss case studies that highlighted the effects of disasters on specific populations. The first breakout panel, moderated by Joelle Simpson, medical director of emergency preparedness at Children's National Hospital, explored the issues brought on by, or exacerbated by, disasters. The second breakout panel, moderated by Heather Beal, founder and president of BLOCKS Inc., explored the effect of disasters on parents and guardians. The third breakout panel, moderated by Ann-Marie Sabrsula, education coordinator and co-administrator for the Arc Westchester Children's School for Early Development, explored the effect of disasters on children with complex or special needs. The fourth breakout panel, moderated by Roberta Lavin, professor at the University of New Mexico College of Nursing, discussed the effect of disasters on unaccompanied minors.

EFFECT ON CHILDREN WITH ISSUES BROUGHT ON BY, OR EXACERBATED BY, DISASTERS

Ensuring Children's Nutrition and Safety During and After Disasters

Scott Needle, chief medical officer at Elica Health Center, discussed nutrition, safety, and environmental concerns for children in disasters. He highlighted the shortcomings of conventional emergency nutrition provisions, which are typically aimed at the needs of adults rather than children and breastfeeding mothers. Mothers, infants, and older children have unique needs related to nutrition, feeding, restrooms, and privacy. Furthermore, these groups have unique needs in terms of supervision, safety, noise, and play spaces, especially in large-scale settings such as mass shelters during hurricanes. He described resources addressing postdisaster family reunification.[1] In the aftermath of hurricanes and floods, there are various safety and environmental hazards that children must be protected from, such as debris, mold, toxins, high temperature, sun exposure, and insects. Similarly, during wildfires and volcano disasters, smoke, soot, and particulate matter can harm the respiratory health of children within a large radius of the disaster. These safety and environmental threats not only put children's health at risk, but they also affect and are connected to children's behavior. Children are curious and generally unable to discern danger in the way that adults can, so children must be carefully supervised during and after disasters to ensure their health and safety. This may be a challenging task during and after disasters, when schools and child care may be closed, and parents are likely to have additional tasks and stressors to manage. Finally, Needle noted that as families return to neighborhoods after disasters, it is important to consider the psychological and environmental needs of children, who often experience a great sense of loss during the disaster experience.

Mental Health and Educational Considerations for Children in Disasters

Tara Powell, associate professor at the University of Illinois at Urbana-Champaign, described the experiences of disaster-affected children. They are often displaced from their homes, separated from loved ones, required to change schools, have unmet basic needs including food and shelter, and face loss of friends, family, and community. Depending on their developmental level, children may experience various emotional reactions and related behaviors after disasters. Young children may experience fear of strangers, separation anxiety, sleep problems, nightmares, posttraumatic play, fussiness, irritability, aggressive behavior, or regression. Children in elementary school may experience behavior changes, refuse to go to school, and have physical complaints. Adolescents may experience drug and alcohol abuse, changes in social interactions, difficulty concentrating, irritability, or other behavior changes. Because mental health is shaped by the convergence of biological, social, and psychological factors, children respond in various ways to their disaster experiences. During and after disasters, children's

---

[1] More information about postdisaster family reunification is available at https://www.fema.gov/media-library-data/1384376663394-eef4a1b4269de14faff40390e4e2f2d3/Post_Disaster_Reunification_of_Children_-_A_Nationwide_Approach.pdf (accessed October 21, 2020) and https://www.aap.org/en-us/Documents/AAP-Reunification-Toolkit.pdf (accessed October 21, 2020).

responses are shaped by their developmental level, physical health, family separation, the level of impact of the disaster event, previous trauma exposure, availability of resources, or perceived threat. She discussed the 3 Es of trauma—the event, the experience, and the effect—each of which can influence the mental health of children during disasters. Most children's mental health does recover from disasters in the long term, she noted.

Powell described the protective factors that can help children overcome their exposure to disasters. These include supportive adults, peer and family relationships, emotional and behavioral regulation, communication skills, and access to basic needs. The social, emotional, and mental health of young people can be supported by

- normalizing their feelings and emotions,
- ensuring that their basic needs are met,
- providing them with accurate and developmentally appropriate information,
- limiting access to media,
- listening to their needs, and
- ensuring that children can engage in interpersonal connection, routines, physical activity, and play.

Powell also explored how school-based interventions can address the social and emotional needs of disaster-affected children. Such interventions may be universal, selective, indicated, or as treatment. Universal interventions may be provided through schools to all children, teaching emotional skills and developing preparedness. Selective programs can be beneficial to any child at risk (e.g., all children in a community that have been exposed to a disaster). These programs are often group based and aimed at reducing short- and long-term risks. Indicated programs are targeted at children experiencing mental health symptoms and may be conducted on the individual level or among small groups. Treatment programs are needed for individual children in need of assistance, such as one-on-one therapy.

PsySTART Pediatric Disaster Mental Health Triage System

Merritt Schreiber, professor of clinical pediatrics in the Department of Pediatrics at the David Geffen School of Medicine at the University of California, Los Angeles, discussed the PsySTART pediatric disaster mental health triage system. He explained that there are various potential trajectories that children may follow after disasters, including resilience pathways (e.g., stress, transitory distress response) and risk pathways (e.g., new incidence disorders). PsySTART is aimed at triaging to stepped care within 30 days of a disaster to interrupt children's progress toward a risk pathway.

Schreiber said that the framework used in PsySTART was adapted from a model developed for the National Child Traumatic Stress Network.[2] The model is focused on integration across disaster systems of care, such as human service organizations, schools, medical settings, families, and other systems of care. Linkage to the appropriate level of care is provided through a rapid triage process. The PsySTART rapid triage model does not require direct questioning of the child, and it shifts the focus of triage from signs of distress to evidence-based risk markers (e.g., children's experiences of being trapped, seeing serious injuries or deaths, thinking that they were going to die, having family members killed or injured, losing their homes, being unaccompanied, and being displaced from their social supports). In some settings, a simplified adverse childhood experiences (ACEs) screening, called ACEs triage, has been implemented. A PsySTART triage smartphone application can be used to conduct the triage process, he added. This triage input process is used to allocate resources based on needs. The application can also provide real-time mapping of population risk and can generate individual referrals based on risk markers. The PsySTART triage system is based on the principle that if these markers and needs are not consistently measured early in the disaster recovery process, then they tend to be missed and go unaddressed. The system has many complex functions and capacities, including mapping, rendering parameter-based risk metrics, generating incident action plans, and creating tools for aligning resources with needs.

Schreiber discussed the use of the PsySTART triage system by the Sonoma County School system in nine underserved rural districts that were significantly affected by wildfire, flooding, and mudslide emergencies. The process began with PsySTART solution-focused triage, screening as many children as possible in the affected area and aligning resources with needs. Next, a 4-hour step 1 intervention of trauma-focused cognitive behavioral therapy was provided via telehealth. If necessary, a 12-hour step 2 intervention of full cognitive behavioral therapy was provided. If these steps can be implemented in the first month after a disaster—the so-called golden month—it may result in the prevention or reduction of posttraumatic stress disorder among disaster-affected children. Sonoma County also used PsySTART to conduct a gap analysis in order to assess and align needs and resources. He added that PsySTART may also be customized to refine the alignment of needs and resources for rapid response to disasters.

---

[2] More information about the National Children's Disaster Health Concept of Operations is available at https://www.aap.org/en-us/Documents/disasters_dpac_NPDCCschreiber.pdf (accessed October 21, 2020).

Research Findings from Hurricane Katrina

Alice Fothergill, Department of Sociology at The University of Vermont, discussed findings from her research on children's experiences of Hurricane Katrina. Her discussion focused on the experiences of children living in poverty before, during, and after the hurricane (Fothergill and Peek, 2015). This research was conducted through a 7-year modified naturalistic study using qualitative interviews conducted with children and various individuals from their families, schools, and communities. To understand children's experiences, the researchers needed to observe the various spheres of children's lives (e.g., family, housing, school, peers, health, extracurricular activities). The study revealed that there is not a definitive endpoint of the effects of Hurricane Katrina.

Three postdisaster trajectories were identified among the children studied, said Fothergill. Children in the declining trajectory experienced simultaneous and ongoing disruptions in their families, schooling, housing, health, and health care. Children in the finding equilibrium trajectory were able to regain or attain stability with mobilization of resources and social support. Children in the fluctuating trajectory experienced a mixed pattern of stability and instability. She noted the connection between economic advantage or disadvantage and the trajectories experienced by children: children of greater economic advantage tended to be in the finding equilibrium or fluctuating trajectories. In their study, they found that all children experienced a decline immediately following the disaster.

Fothergill presented three vignettes that exemplified the three trajectories. The declining trajectory reveals the effect of cumulative vulnerability (i.e., the overall effect of numerous preexisting vulnerabilities when a disaster occurs). Most children on the finding equilibrium trajectory had access to resources. However, Fothergill shared a nontypical example of a child who did not have access to resources prior to Hurricane Katrina but who benefited from resource mobilization after the hurricane. Through linkages to advocates, this child and her family were able to obtain housing, mental health care, mentoring, and other forms of assistance. Her family had no resources before the storm, so she would not have been expected to find equilibrium after losing everything in Hurricane Katrina. The fact that she found equilibrium shows the importance of resource mobilization as part of the disaster response, said Fothergill.

She described two patterns in the fluctuating trajectory: multiple spheres in flux and all spheres simultaneously in flux. She shared an example of two siblings who experienced a fluctuating trajectory with all spheres simultaneously in flux, noting that this case reveals the importance of adult "anchors." Anchors are adults in a child's life who prevent the children from "falling through the cracks" as they experience fluctuations in their life spheres. They may include older siblings, grandparents, or other adults to whom they are socially connected.

Social engagement is another key factor for children who are in flux; social engagement may be the means through which children find their adult anchors (e.g., coaches, teachers). Fothergill highlighted the capacity of children to help one another as well as helping adults. Children have voices and problem-solving skills that should be involved in disaster recovery efforts to whatever extent possible. She also noted the importance of housing and returning to school for children's recovery. While returning to school was an essential part of recovery—offering routine, stability, food, and links to other resources—children recovering from disasters also need accommodations and assistance to return to school. During Hurricane Katrina, housing programs of every kind, from many organizations, were shown to be highly beneficial to the child recipients of those programs. This illustrates how a web of mobilized resources and services are needed to help children find equilibrium after a disaster, said Fothergill.

EFFECT OF DISASTERS ON PARENTS AND GUARDIANS

Disaster Effects on Parents, Caregivers, and Child Care

Holly Nett, director of Child Care Emergency Partnerships at Child Care Aware of America, discussed how disasters can affect parents, caregivers, and child care. Child Care Aware of America is a national membership-based nonprofit focusing exclusively on child care. It serves as a leading voice in the United States advocating for child care system improvement, working with more than 600 state and local child care resource and referral agencies to help ensure that families have access to high-quality and affordable child care. These organizations typically offer child care program referrals, consumer education, and financial assistance for families and professional development and technical assistance for child care program staff, along with advocacy on early childhood issues, recruitment and retention of programs in communities, and partnership building.

Nett commented that during disasters, children under 5 years of age are among the most vulnerable. Children of this age are often separated from their families when a disaster strikes because they are in child care settings. Child care programs are especially vulnerable to disasters because children are unable to protect themselves and are reliant on their child care providers to ensure their safety. In times of calm and as well as during disasters, Child Care Aware of America uses its relationships, data, and technology to help communities understand the landscape of child care before, during, and after an emergency. It focuses its efforts on building preparedness, determining needs, mapping the effects of emergencies, and locating temporary care during recovery. Given the inevitability of disasters, a well-prepared child care workforce is necessary to ensure children's safety during an emergency, she noted. Parents must have a great deal of trust in their children's health care providers, which takes on a new dimension in the context of disasters. Well-trained caregivers are more likely to be able to provide needed emotional and physical support to children during disasters.

Child Care Aware of America has also been working to address the research gap on child care emergency preparedness for infants and toddlers, said Nett. In 2018, it surveyed early learning professionals to develop evacuation recommendations for children during emergencies.[3] Nearly 20 percent of survey respondents reported that they have had to evacuate infants or toddlers because of an emergency, such as fire, smoke, gas leaks or smells, and severe weather. These kinds of emergencies are an area of focus because of infants' and toddlers' unique reliance on caregivers for physical, nutritional, and emotional support; their limited communication abilities; their limited mobility; and their reliance on caregivers for protection from harm.

Nett also described the effects of disasters on child care since 2012. In disasters such as Superstorm Sandy, flooding in Louisiana, Hurricane Harvey, and California wildfires, numerous child care facilities reported damages and were forced to close because of these disasters. These damages and closures each displaced many children who were in need of child care, and the shortage of child care can hinder communities' ability to recover from disasters. Child care resource and referral agencies and partners can play a major role in recovery by helping to funnel resources to communities in need of child care, she added. This kind of response requires that relationships be in place prior to disasters, however. Recognizing that emergency preparedness, response, and recovery is vital to the well-being of children, families, and communities, Child Care Aware of America's emergency preparedness team is committed to providing resources to child care resource and referral agencies and partnering agencies to support the needs of the child care sector before, during, and after emergencies.[4]

Issues for Parents and Guardians: Housing and Mental Health

Jonathan Sury, National Center for Disaster Preparedness, discussed issues for parents and guardians related to housing and mental health and disasters. He described the evolving disaster landscape. Factors such as

---

[3] More information about the Child Care Aware of America 2018 survey is available at https://info.childcareaware.org/blog/child-care-prepare-infant-toddler-emergency-evacuation (accessed April 6, 2021).

[4] More information about the Child Care Aware of America's emergency preparedness efforts is available at https://ChildCarePrepare.org (accessed October 21, 2020).

emerging infectious diseases, extreme weather events, technological and human-made disasters, and information overload have introduced new concerns and added complexity to communications about disasters in ways that affect planning.

Sury highlighted several themes from research about Hurricane Katrina, Superstorm Sandy, Hurricane Florence, and Hurricane Maria. In communities most affected by these disasters, there were preexisting housing crises—characterized by high-risk housing, poor mitigation, and housing policies—and reconstruction and rebuilding in these communities has been slow, often owing to the lack of resources. These communities have also been affected by mental health issues, with the mental health of parents and guardians having a great effect on the mental health of children after disasters. He noted that trusted child-serving institutions are necessary for resuming economic activity after most disasters.

Sury presented a socioeconomic model of recovery that identified five predictors of postdisaster recovery: housing stability, stable economic resources, good mental health, good physical health, and positive social role adaptation (Abramson et al., 2010). He highlighted the effect of financial stressors on postdisaster recovery. After Superstorm Sandy, residents who suffered major structural damage were 2.5 times as likely to have difficulty affording rent, bills, mortgage, food, or transportation, regardless of income. Furthermore, residents living in poverty were 6.7 times as likely to have difficulty paying bills. These financial stressors translate into a decrease in mental health, he noted. In this research, housing damage, prior history of depression, and identifying as Hispanic were found to be positive predictors of posttraumatic stress disorder. He discussed unpublished data collected from households affected by Hurricane Harvey, which indicate that 40 percent of homes with children in 2017 still needed to repair damage caused by the hurricane. Moreover, 27 percent of the homes surveyed needed housing assistance, 37 percent of heads of household respondents reported that their own lives were still disrupted by the hurricane, and 60 percent of respondents said that their households had still not recovered from the hurricane. He also presented findings from a study on housing stability after Hurricane Katrina, which demonstrates the connections between housing instability and mental health disability, poor sense of community, inadequate social support, worse academic performance among children, and emotional problems among children.

Sury called for the following:

- Investing in long-term financial support for community-based organizations to offer housing repair and extend the duration of housing assistance programs,
- Building capacity among parents and guardians so they may better serve as resilient buffers for their children, and

- Formally integrate local emergency management, licensing, and social services for child-focused preparedness issues (e.g., staff, funding), perhaps including child-specific community liaisons.

He advocated for uniting preparedness planning guidance and technical and financial assistance for child care centers, particularly in Puerto Rico. He also noted that foster families generally are not required to develop their own household disaster plans, and they often require technical assistance to create such plans. Finally, he underscored the importance of connecting with, and listening to, the needs of affected communities.

Effects of Disasters on Parents and Guardians

C. J. Huff, educator and child advocate, shared his personal experience working as a part of numerous disaster responses and discussed the key role of schools as part of postdisaster recovery efforts. School systems are essential during crises, he said. They offer familiar environments, trusted relationships, access to services and support, and other valuable resources. These supports are particularly important for families and children with access and functional needs, resource-challenged families, and undocumented families. School systems that are affected by disasters face the challenge of adapting to find ways to continue to deliver school services, such as individual education plans, assistive devices, and curricula. For instance, the COVID-19 pandemic has forced schools to adapt their approach to each of these service types; these adaptations have put additional stress on parents and their children throughout the pandemic. Furthermore, the increased stresses experienced by parents during disasters often change family dynamics and may result in child abuse.

He emphasized the importance of emergency operations planning, keeping digital records, maintaining up-to-date contact information, ensuring continuity of learning planning, and developing community partnerships. All of these efforts can help schools navigate unexpected situations that arise during and after disasters, he noted. He added that other community needs should also be considered in advance of disasters, such as creating children and youth task forces, mapping resources, creating mutual aid agreements, and establishing university partnerships. At the federal level, he suggested creating assistive device inventories in advance of disasters, establishing philanthropic partnerships, creating resource databases, increasing funding for the School Emergency Response to Violence program,[5] and placing disaster case managers in schools.

---

[5] More information about the School Emergency Response to Violence program is available at https://www2.ed.gov/programs/dvppserv/index.html (accessed April 6, 2020).

Discussion

Beal asked about data that demonstrate the effect of the loss of child care on disaster recovery. Nett said that there is much anecdotal evidence about the child care struggles of communities during disaster recovery, but more research is needed. Beal also asked whether the lessons learned during the COVID-19 pandemic may inform future responses to disasters. Huff said that schools' COVID-19 responses have highlighted issues of equity, particularly in rural areas where connectivity is limited. Predisaster planning and educator training can enable schools to respond to disasters effectively. Furthermore, parent engagement is invaluable for supporting instruction, especially as online instruction has become the new norm during the COVID-19 pandemic response, he added.

Beal asked whether a postdisaster mental health program that is oriented to the family or the child care provider could help to address the mental health issues that arise during and after disasters. Sury replied that like all disaster response programs, trauma-informed communities should be established in advance of disasters. He cited a cadre of Community Resilience Model trainers in South Carolina who teach a wide range of professionals in all public sectors to equip them with a trauma-informed approach to interacting with their communities. People who may interact with children who have experienced a disaster should also receive training in psychological first aid, he added. However, implementing these models may give rise to resource allocation issues. He shared his experience with working in a community to create a mental health response plan. He noted that engaging all relevant stakeholders for such efforts is challenging, but a community plan may be critical for adequately providing a sustained mental health response to disasters, especially one that can address both acute and chronic mental health challenges.

Acknowledging the critical roles of child care, schools, mental health support, and housing stability for disaster recovery, Beal asked which other systems should be established and maintained prior to disasters to ensure adequate disaster recovery. Nett said that partnerships should be established and maintained to help support disaster planning systems; strong partnerships also help to ensure that resources can be mobilized during disasters. Sury said that local emergency management institutions are consistently understaffed and underresourced, often without any specific plans for children. Increasing funding and creating child-specific emergency planning positions and institutions would help to connect all of the key factors discussed by the panel and ensure that planning for disasters—including planning for the needs of children—is ongoing during "blue sky times." Huff remarked that "cash is king:" during emergencies, cash funds should be available to address needs as they arise. He reiterated that preexisting and well-maintained relationships in communities are the key to community resilience. By routinely convening, planning, and problem solving for disasters and other issues, community groups can "exercise their reliance muscles" so that they can be harnessed during disasters. Sury added that communities often need technical assistance to establish their disaster response plans.

Beal asked whether a federally funded mandate for children and youth task forces would be an appropriate vehicle to realize the plans and systems advocated by the panelists. Huff said that the investment into such task forces is primarily directed toward training and the establishment of frameworks. With each disaster and community being different, children and youth task forces should be designed to build on the unique strengths within each community. Thus, a federal mandate for children and youth task forces may not be warranted, but state-level encouragement of the creation of such task forces may be beneficial. In either case, the success of children and youth task forces depends on the leadership capacity in each community, he added. Sury said that tapping into preexisting community structures for any purpose would be helpful. Using community champions who have existing relationships, credibility, and convening power within the community has been shown to be an effective approach.

EFFECT OF DISASTERS ON CHILDREN WITH COMPLEX OR SPECIAL NEEDS

Needs of Students with Disabilities and Their Families During Disasters

Kate Moran and Carmen Sanchez, education program specialists at the Department of Education, shared the experiences of students with disabilities and their families during disasters. Moran shared images from Hurricane Maria depicting the destruction of roads, homes, and infrastructure and the barriers that these disruptions created for individuals with special needs. She explained that power and transportation disruptions caused difficulties for individuals who relied on wheelchairs and elevators for mobility. Similarly, individuals who relied on oxygen tanks were put at risk by infrastructure disruptions. In some cases, disaster responders have been unable to access the homes of individuals who were known to need assistance because of disruptions and damage caused by disasters. The Office of Special Education Programs (OSEP) provides disaster support including food items, durable medical equipment, breathing equipment, feeding equipment, mobility equipment, and translators to assist those with special communication needs (e.g., deaf individuals). Moran explained that OSEP works with state governments to create systems to address the loss of paper documents during disasters and the transference of data into electronic record systems. Their office plays a role in facilitating interagency collaboration by connecting disability specialists from various agencies during disaster response. This facilitating role is helpful in identifying where additional support is needed for those with special needs.

Sanchez discussed the discretionary grants provided through OSEP. Grants are given to nonprofit parent organizations and are intended to help families of children with disabilities to learn about their rights and to work with their schools and educators to provide for the needs of children with disabilities. She emphasized that for children with special needs, it is often difficult to separate their educational needs from their health needs or other fundamental needs. These grants are provided on a 5-year cycle, but many grantees have held their grants for 30 years or more. These grantees have become resource hubs, serving as "one-stop shops" for the families of children with special needs. Currently, 96 centers are supported by these grants, and a tight-knit community has been formed among these grantees.

One national center is funded by these grants, the Center for Parent Information and Resources,[6] along with four regional centers. These national and regional technical assistance centers are important in disaster response, especially for families with children with special needs who need to relocate across states during a disaster. These national and regional centers help to facilitate the transition process and ensure that parent centers are sharing information. For instance, these centers were critical for facilitating the transitions of many families from Louisiana to Texas during Hurricane Katrina.

Sanchez shared a story of a woman in Puerto Rico who was trapped with her teenage son after Hurricane Maria. Her son used an electric wheelchair and required pureed food. She struggled to find food for her son, but the parent information center in Puerto Rico—which was funded by OSEP grants—was closed because of hurricane damage. The mother was able to contact a parent center in New Jersey and received relief through the actions of various individuals within the national network of parent centers. Sanchez added that many families with children with special needs who moved from Puerto Rico to Florida or other states used the network of parent centers to facilitate their transition. She noted that Fairfax, Virginia, has created a special needs emergency registry that allows any person to register themself or a family member that has special needs so that during an emergency, disaster responders know the location and specific needs of those registrants in advance.

---

[6] Sanchez explained that the Center for Parent Information and Resources has strategically assembled resources for parents in response to the COVID-19 pandemic. More information is available at https://www.parentcenterhub.org (accessed October 22, 2020).

Psychological and Social Effects of Disasters on Children and Youth with Disabilities

Laura Stough, associate professor and assistant director of the Center on Disability and Development at Texas A&M University, noted that research on individuals with disabilities and special health care needs during disasters has been increasing since the aftermath of Hurricane Katrina. However, this body of research is still limited and is primarily focused on adults rather than children and youth (Stough and Kelman, 2018). The evidence available, however, confirms that those with disabilities are disproportionately affected by disasters. They experience higher mortality rates and higher degrees of property loss. People with disabilities tend to be equally prepared for disasters as those without disabilities, but persons with disabilities may (1) have greater need for support during evacuation and sheltering, (2) require more intensive case management during recovery periods, and (3) take longer to recover from disasters.

Approximately 20 percent of U.S. children under 18 years of age have special health care needs, said Stough (HRSA Maternal & Child Health Bureau, 2020). Many children with disabilities have difficulties related to mobility, communication, or learning. Children with disabilities and their families often rely on education and community supports that can be disrupted in disasters (Peek and Stough, 2010). However, studies have found that levels of emergency preparedness vary among families with children with special health care needs (Baker and Baker, 2010; Baker and Cormier, 2013; Wolf-Fordham et al., 2015). Small-scale public health interventions have been successful in helping families prepare for emergencies (Bagwell et al., 2016), but families of children with disabilities may require tailored disaster information to best meet their needs (Hipper et al., 2018). She remarked that when rapid evacuation is required, preparedness for children with disabilities is critical.

Stough discussed the experiences of children who were exposed to the California wildfires in 2017.[7] Parents of these children did not receive preparedness information or evacuation support specific to disability-related needs. Families encountered difficulties in evacuating children with disabilities along with their durable medical equipment and assistive technology. Parents often evacuated alone with their children and, after evacuating, they often faced difficulties in accommodating disability-related needs as they transitioned to multiple temporary housing situations. These families encountered psychological stresses associated with these experiences, but the postdisaster psychological supports available were not adapted for chil-

---

[7] More information about children with special health care needs being evacuated during wildfires is available at https://hazards.colorado.edu/news/research-counts/evacuating-under-fire-children-with-special-healthcare-needs-in-disaster (accessed October 22, 2020).

dren with disabilities. More collaboration is needed among voluntary agencies, disability organizations, and health care providers to deliver needed supplies, equipment, and support during and after emergencies, she said.

Few studies have looked at the psychological experiences of children with disabilities experiencing disasters (Stough et al., 2017). However, people with developmental disabilities may have difficulties when encountering unusual or unexpected stimuli, which often occur in emergency situations. Furthermore, there has been a lack of interventions adapted for children with cognitive disabilities or autism spectrum disorder. This is concerning, Stough said, given that children with developmental disabilities experience disproportionate trauma exposure. She called for trauma-informed, school-based measures to address these concerns. She said that schools have a responsibility to ensure whole community drills, evacuation plans, and sheltering in place to ensure the safety of students with disabilities. However, the needs of children with disabilities are often excluded in school disaster planning (Fifolt et al., 2017), and students with disabilities are often excluded in disaster education efforts (Boon et al., 2014; Stough et al., 2020). Several studies have demonstrated that students with disabilities can effectively participate in disaster education with curricular modifications (Ronoh et al., 2015a,b).

Despite being affected by disasters themselves, teachers provide essential support to students and their families throughout all phases of disasters, said Stough. Teachers' roles often expand during disasters to include instrumental and psychological supports. For instance, special education teachers may provide support even when schools are closed and students have been displaced from their school districts (McAdams Ducy and Stough, 2011). School personnel need to be well trained and knowledgeable across school contexts, said Stough (Stough et al., 2020). She added that the effects of disasters on school personnel themselves must be considered postdisaster when schools begin reopening and must rely on these personnel in order to resume instruction.

Finally, Stough discussed the roles of voluntary and nonprofit organizations in disaster response. The specific needs of people with disabilities are often ignored or overlooked by volunteers providing disaster response, and volunteers are often not trained to identify and assist individuals with disabilities (International Federation of Red Cross and Red Crescent Societies, 2007). Few of the volunteer organizations active in disasters that are part of the national response framework focus specifically on the needs of persons with disabilities, she added. However, disability-related organizations have been participating more actively in issues surrounding emergency management and disaster risk reduction. She suggested that this increased interest by disability organizations may be attributable, at least in part, to the COVID-19 pandemic and the threat posed by the pandemic to individuals with developmental disabilities. Finally, she pointed out that disability-related organizations are often not connected with local emergency management.

Discussion

Sabrsula asked whether any initiatives are under way to fill the gaps in addressing the long-term psychological effects of disasters on students with special needs. Stough said that there is a lack of modified psychological treatments for students with intellectual disabilities; she pointed out that these students are often at a greater risk of experiencing trauma, even outside of the disaster context.

Sabrsula asked whether any new efforts are under way to promote training for disaster response. Moran said that various forms of training are available that include elements of support strategies, particularly in the context of the COVID-19 pandemic. Sanchez said that the Center for Parent Information and Resources has created a webpage to direct parents to places that offer training on trauma-informed care. She mentioned two centers that focus on behavior: the Center on Positive Behavioral Interventions and Supports has begun working with trauma,[8] and the National Center for Pyramid Model Innovations addresses behavior among younger children.[9] Moran shared a link to the Early Childhood Technical Assistance Center website, which offers resources on disaster planning and trauma response.[10] Stough explained that these and other related resources are valuable, but none of those resources or interventions are tailored to address the specific needs of children with preexisting disabilities and complex health care needs. For instance, many of these children express depression or anxiety through behavior, but many school counselors are not trained to interpret these behaviors as expressions of anxiety, trauma, or grief.

Sabrsula asked how children with disabilities can be supported while living in shelters. Moran replied that it may be possible to work with those children and their families through cooperation with the Federal Emergency Management Agency (FEMA). She suggested that disability integration specialists are often connected to FEMA, city governments, and other agencies. Thus, such specialists are likely the best point of access for assisting families with children with disabilities living in shelters.

---

[8] More information about the Center on Positive Behavioral Interventions and Supports is available at https://www.pbis.org (accessed October 22, 2020).

[9] More information about the National Center for Pyramid Model Innovations is available at https://challengingbehavior.cbcs.usf.edu/index.html (accessed October 22, 2020).

[10] More information about disaster planning and trauma response is available at https://ectacenter.org/topics/disaster/disaster.asp (accessed October 22, 2020).

EFFECT OF DISASTERS ON UNACCOMPANIED MINORS

Disasters and Unaccompanied Minors

Patricia Frost, vice chair of the National Pediatric Disaster Coalition, discussed the effects that disasters have on unaccompanied minors. If children become unaccompanied minors during disasters, they may experience lifelong consequences. While policy makers are often aware of fault lines, flood zones, or other environmental risk factors, they are often unaware of community risk factors and resources available to address them. Better awareness of community risks, including awareness of the location of at-risk children, is important for disaster preparedness.

Frost noted that the disaster response system is geared toward response rather than addressing short-term and long-term consequences. The multisectoral rescue chain—beginning at the impact zone and extending through evacuation processes and into hospitals—is often chaotic and involves multiple handoffs. This chain puts children at risk of being lost in the system, especially during no-notice and short-notice events.

Hurricane Katrina was emblematic of these challenges and brought attention to the effects of disasters on unaccompanied minors, said Frost. She cited the case of Cortez Stewart, who was not reunited with her family until 6 months after the hurricane. During Hurricane Katrina, myriad systematic breakdowns, coupled with a lack of infrastructure, made it difficult for families to keep their children with them through the response and recovery processes. Additionally, many families experienced delays in evacuation and in receiving information that affected their ability to keep their children with them. During Hurricane Katrina, many unaccompanied minors were sent to mass shelters; some of those minors arrived in the company of nonguardian adults, at least one of whom was later found to be a sexual predator. Furthermore, foster care services struggled to track and manage their more than 500 foster children, and law enforcement lost track of numerous sexual offenders during that period. Frost shared several examples of children who underwent traumatic experiences during Hurricane Katrina after being separated from their families.

Superstorm Sandy raised similar concerns about unaccompanied minors, said Frost. In New York City, 230 homeless shelters were lost because of storm surges and 300 homeless families had to be relocated. Programs for homeless youth and for lesbian, gay, bisexual, and transgender youth were also disproportionately affected by the storm. These vulnerable individuals had a desperate need to access already crowded emergency shelters. During the storm, nearly 8,700 students were dislocated to live in shelters, hotels, or with other families. Families in poverty were found to have a higher risk of being separated, she noted.

In 2018, wildfires in Paradise, California, required evacuations followed by multiple relocations of shelters owing to the rapid advancement of fires. Many children who were evacuated during this disaster were separated or at risk of being separated from their families, said Frost. In one case, a school bus driver took the initiative to evacuate 22 students directly from an elementary school without having any opportunity to contact these children's families. Frost noted that although there are best practices for reunification, the ultimate aim should be to prevent family separation by implementing proper infrastructure, offering training, ensuring coordination, and providing other necessary resources.[11]

Programs for Homeless and Runaway Youth and Parents

Jeff Daniels, program manager of the Runaway and Homeless Youth Program at the Administration for Children and Families (ACF), gave an overview of the programs operated by the program. It provides discretionary funds to grantees for street outreach, basic center outreach, transitional living programs, and maternity group homes.

Street outreach programs support work with homeless, runaway, and street youth to assist them in finding stable housing and accessing services,[12] said Daniels. These programs focus on developing relationships between outreach workers and young people that allow them to rebuild connections with caring adults. The programs are also aimed at preventing sexual exploitation and abuse of youth on the streets. Street outreach services include education and outreach, emergency shelter access, survival aid, treatment and counseling, crisis intervention, and follow-up support.

ACF's Basic Center program creates and strengthens community-based programs that meet the immediate needs of runaway and homeless youth under 18 years of age. These programs also aim to reunite young people with their families or locate appropriate alternative placements, said Daniels. Basic Center program services include up to 21 days of shelter, food, clothing, medical care, crisis intervention, recreation programs, aftercare services, and counseling for individuals, groups, and families. Transitional living program services are provided to older homeless youth, with supporting projects that provide long-term residential services to

---

[11] More information about postdisaster family reunification is available at https://www.fema.gov/media-library-data/1384376663394-eef4a1b4269de14faff40390e4e2f2d3/Post_Disaster_Reunification_of_Children_-_A_Nationwide_Approach.pdf (accessed October 21, 2020) and https://www.aap.org/en-us/Documents/AAP-Reunification-Toolkit.pdf (accessed October 21, 2020).

[12] Daniels explained that "runaway youth" are defined as youth who purposely leave their home, while "homeless youth" can describe a person 22 years of age or younger who has become homeless under certain circumstances through no fault of their own.

homeless young people. Young people aged 16–22 years are eligible for these programs. Living accommodations may include host family homes, group homes, maternity group homes, or supervised apartments owned by the program or rented in the community.

Transitional living programs offer or provide referrals to additional services, including safe and stable living accommodations, basic life skills building, educational opportunities, job attainment services, mental health care, and physical health care. Maternity group homes for pregnant youth and parenting youth programs support homeless pregnant or parenting young people (aged 16–22 years) along with their dependent children. In addition to the services offered by transitional living programs, maternity group home programs offer parenting skills, child development services, family budgeting, and health and nutrition services, said Daniels.

Daniels explained that emergency preparedness planning was critical for managing the Paradise wildfire disaster in 2018. Approximately 22,000 individuals were displaced by the fires, but within hours of the evacuation, one ACF grantee organization in Paradise had accounted for all staff and children managed by the program. Additionally, the organization was able to provide temporary housing for staff whose homes were destroyed by the wildfires.

Human Trafficking Identification and Responses in Disaster Contexts

Leanne McCallum, task force coordinator at the Greater New Orleans Human Trafficking Task Force, discussed frameworks for understanding the vulnerabilities of unaccompanied minors to human trafficking in the postdisaster context. Sex trafficking is defined as the recruitment, harboring, transportation, provision, obtaining, patronizing, or soliciting of a person for the purposes of a commercial sex act, in which the commercial sex act is induced by force, fraud, or coercion, or in which the person induced to perform such an act has not attained 18 years of age (22 USC § 7102). Labor trafficking is the recruitment, harboring, transportation, provision, or obtaining of a person for labor or services, through the use of force, fraud, or coercion for the purposes of subjection to involuntary servitude, peonage, debt bondage, or slavery (22 USC § 7102).

Unaccompanied minors are vulnerable to both sex trafficking and labor trafficking, said McCallum. In disaster contexts, some young people participate in survival sex by trading commercial sex acts for things of value (e.g., food, protection, shelter, other basic needs). As defined in the context of sex and labor trafficking, force, fraud, or coercion may include lack of mobility, debt bondage, document confiscation, recruitment fraud, lack of payment, physical or sexual abuse, threats of violence or retribution, long hours without reprieve, or the inability to walk away.

A person's inability to walk away is the primary distinguishing factor of trafficking, she added.

Young people face particular vulnerabilities during disasters that put them at risk of becoming victims of trafficking:

- Risk of homelessness or displacement;
- Loss of jobs or other ways of making money;
- Isolation;
- Reliance on others for basic needs like food, water, and shelter;
- Lack of protection from law enforcement or labor rights agencies;
- Suspension of some labor protection systems;
- Limited interactions with mandated reporters or safe figures; and
- Other cultural factors.

Certain children are highly vulnerable to trafficking during the postdisaster period, including those without parental care or who are living on their own, living in foster care, living with mental or physical disabilities, living with special needs, and children who are members of marginalized groups.

McCallum shared lessons learned from disasters in which child trafficking was discovered. Common themes from trafficking after these disasters included displacement and movement of people as a condition in which trafficking occurred, false promises made to victims, damage to homes and livelihoods causing vulnerability to trafficking, the presence of vulnerabilities before the disaster, and the use of false adoptions for trafficking. She added that child marriage—a form of trafficking—may also increase during postdisaster periods.

National Center for Missing & Exploited Children

Joy Paluska, program manager in the disaster preparedness and response program at the National Center for Missing & Exploited Children (NCMEC), described the history of NCMEC, a nonprofit nongovernmental organization established in 1984 that receives approximately 70 percent of its funding from the Department of Justice. NCMEC was established after its founding members observed that there was no system in place for searching for missing children in the United States. NCMEC's mission is to find missing children, reduce child sexual exploitation, and prevent future victimization. NCMEC comprises a wide variety of service and programs that liaise with various law enforcement and government agencies.

A missing child is defined as a person who has not yet reached 18 years of age whose whereabouts are unknown to a legal guardian (42 USC § 5772), said Paluska. A separated child is a child who is separated from both parents or from their previous legal or customary primary caregiver, but not necessarily from other relatives. Unaccompanied children are children who have been separated from both parents and other relatives and are not being cared for by an adult who, by law or custom, is responsible for doing so.[13]

Paluska described NCMEC's role in Hurricane Katrina, explaining that NCMEC's federal mandate has expanded as NCMEC has demonstrated additional capacities related to helping missing children. After Hurricane Katrina, NCMEC provided field support to help locate missing children and family members and identify unaccompanied minors. NCMEC resolved 5,192 missing children cases reported to NCMEC after Hurricane Katrina. NCMEC also established a hotline to handle incoming calls about missing children, ultimately handling 34,045 such calls. NCMEC now operates the federally mandated National Emergency Child Locator Center, which is a call center that connects to NCMEC's 24/7 hotline.

More than 1.5 million people were evacuated during the Hurricane Katrina disasters, including 200,000 children, said Paluska. The evacuation was conducted with no prior planning for vulnerable populations, including children—many of whom were separated from their families. For example, children were put on evacuation buses without their parents and without any tracking system in place; the buses departed in varying directions toward state-managed emergency shelters. In 2006, the Post-Katrina Emergency Management Reform Act included plans to better prepare recovery teams to reunify families. Photographs are typically the quickest way to locate missing individuals, said Paluska. However, in 2005, photos of missing individuals were not often readily available, especially during disasters.

In the years since Hurricane Katrina, improvements in disaster preparedness, technology, and other systems may help to ensure that many of the challenges related to unaccompanied minors that arose during that disaster will be less severe in future disasters, said Paluska. Currently, NCMEC has a strong focus on disaster preparedness and works in coordination with FEMA, the Salvation Army, and the American Red Cross. NCMEC missing children specialists work as FEMA contractors, assisting with issues related to unaccompanied and missing children during disasters. She added that NCMEC operates an unaccompanied minors registry, a national data collection tool used to facilitate the tracking and reunification of unaccompanied minors, expedite the reunification of unaccompanied

---

[13] Separated child and unaccompanied child are defined as per FEMA's postdisaster family reunification approach. More information about postdisaster family reunification is available at https://www.fema.gov/media-library-data/1384376663394-eef4a1b4269de-14faff40390e4e2f2d3/Post_Disaster_Reunification_of_Children_-_A_Nationwide_Approach.pdf (accessed October 21, 2020).

minors with their families, and provide reports back to law enforcement and reunification staff.[14]

Discussion

Lavin asked about gaps in the handling of unaccompanied minors and how they might be addressed. Frost said that many first responders and persons in emergency management roles are not aware of available disaster management and reunification resources and do not fully understand how those resources would connect to their work during a disaster. Much work remains to be done to promote awareness of such resources and ensure adequate disaster preparedness, she added. Daniels said that FEMA has an emergency operation plan that organizations can use for disaster preparedness; it identifies the critical elements of all emergencies and has some information related to unaccompanied minors.

Lavin remarked that children tend to have common core needs during disasters, but children who are being exploited before disasters and youth who are homeless before disasters are especially vulnerable during disasters. Paluska said that disasters uproot individuals' lives and often lead individuals to make decisions that they otherwise might not—for example, during disasters, vulnerable children have a heightened risk of being trafficked. McCallum said that the commercial component distinguishes trafficking from other forms of abuse. Abusers may recruit or try to capitalize on the disaster. For instance, during the post–Hurricane Katrina period, some individuals were forced to do construction labor in unsafe conditions because they had no other way to obtain money or shelter. During that period, child sex abuse and sex trafficking were also occurring among children who became vulnerable because they were abruptly separated from their guardians and others who could identify them as victims. She said that in disaster contexts, the separation of vulnerable individuals from those who would be able to identify them as victims is a major contributing factor to increases in trafficking and abuse.

Lavin asked about the challenges to be addressed in meeting the needs of homeless and missing youth, especially during disasters. Paluska said that most missing youth recorded by NCMEC are "endangered runaways." These individuals are highly vulnerable to exploitation and lack the protection and support networks that might otherwise prevent them from being exploited. Daniels noted that the organization that successfully accounted for its youth and staff during the 2018 Paradise wildfires benefited greatly from the preparation and action of its emergency preparedness team. He

_____
[14] More information about NCMEC's unaccompanied minors registry is available at http://umr.missingkids.org (accessed October 23, 2020).

said that ensuring accountability and safety during emergencies requires communicating, having resources and assets in place in advance, assigning specific staff responsibilities, and planning in advance. He noted that street outreach is another way to help ensure the safety of homeless and unaccompanied minors. In addition to drop-in centers, street outreach helps organizations ensure the safety of youth in their communities. Street outreach varies by community and geography, he added. In some areas, street outreach entails venturing into the forest where homeless youth are living. Efforts should be proactive in seeking out these youth rather than relying on youth in need to come to drop-in centers for help, he said.

Paluska emphasized the need for preparedness, because having plans in place in advance of a crisis is invaluable for ensuring the safety of youth during disasters. Frost said that FEMA Emergency Support Functions (ESFs) 6 and 8 are closely tied to supporting children.[15] However, greater dialogue should be facilitated between health and human resources actors and health care system actors, as these systems operate separately in many ways. Daniels said that planning is key, invoking the adage that "failing to plan is a plan to fail." Disaster planning should take a holistic approach that accounts for all community needs and resources, he added. McCallum called for integrating antitrafficking and domestic violence responses into postdisaster plans in order to help save lives during the disaster response period.

---

[15] More information about ESFs 6 and 8 is available at https://www.fema.gov/pdf/emergency/nrf/nrf-esf-06.pdf (accessed October 23, 2020) and https://www.fema.gov/pdf/emergency/nrf/nrf-esf-08.pdf (accessed October 23, 2020).

6

Workshop Reflections

During the final session, workshop planning committee members shared their reflections on the workshop presentations and discussions. Topics included strengthening child care infrastructure, placing the needs of vulnerable populations in the center of disaster preparation efforts, resource and data accessibility, interdisciplinary collaboration, educating children about disaster preparedness, considerations of the effects of trauma, and monitoring and evaluating response and recovery efforts. Panelists included Heather Beal, founder and president of BLOCKS Inc.; Sherlita Amler, commissioner of the Westchester County, New York, Department of Health; Joelle Simpson, medical director of emergency preparedness at Children's National Hospital; and Tarah Somers, regional director, Region 1 of the Agency for Toxic Substances and Disease Registry. The discussion was moderated by Roberta Lavin, professor at the University of New Mexico College of Nursing.

CLOSING REFLECTIONS ON THE WORKSHOP

In moderating the breakout session on the effect of disasters on parents and guardians, Beal said that themes surfaced related to the criticality of infrastructure that supports children. Availability of child care and schools after a disaster was highlighted, as this restores a routine for children, enables parents and guardians to return to work and rebuild their community, and gives families a sense of normalcy. The group also discussed the need for a return to stable housing as quickly as possible postdisaster, as unstable housing is a stressor for parents and guardians that in turn affects children and their ability to recover.

Amler reflected that a focus on children is the best approach to improving disaster preparation efforts. She noted that gaps in existing research, funding, support, and evidence-based interventions need to be addressed. Planning should occur at the local level—because disasters begin and end locally—but leadership is needed at all levels. Amler said that children can be empowered with an understanding of risks and protective actions that they can take, even if those actions are small. This knowledge enables children to remain calm, be less anxious, and participate actively and competently during an emergency (e.g., making their own go bag). She added that this knowledge may also encourage a lifelong interest in preparedness.

Furthermore, she suggested that the entire family should be considered in disaster preparation and response and that programs should work to build resiliency in both children and adults. This cannot be done in isolation and requires agencies to have a multigenerational approach. Professionals should integrate knowledge about the effect of childhood trauma into the development of policies and procedures. Lastly, she suggested enhancing mental health support through programs such as the psychological first aid program, which can help children learn to cope with the effects of trauma and enable them to successfully navigate difficult circumstances.[1]

Simpson's main lesson was the importance of interweaving services for children, including the education system, health care system, social services, and case management. Much good work is being done and many lessons have been learned since Hurricane Katrina, but there is a need to be more thoughtful about the data that inform services in order to avoid duplicative work and to enhance one another's efforts to serve children and the adults caring for them. Somers emphasized the importance of groups with ongoing operations in communities having access to state and federal programs and services when disasters strike. Additionally, ongoing and continued collaboration across sectors is needed, as this connects the emergency response sector to the early care and education sector before a disaster. This connection then facilitates work on projects and solving problems after a disaster, enabling sectors to move forward together.

STRENGTHENING SUPPORT FOR CHILDREN AND YOUTH IN DISASTERS

Strengthening Critical Child Care Infrastructure

Lavin said that years ago, while working on critical infrastructure for public health and health care, she and colleagues conducted an exhaustive

---

[1] More information about psychological first aid is available at https://www.nctsn.org/treatments-and-practices/psychological-first-aid-and-skills-for-psychological-recovery/about-pfa (accessed October 23, 2020).

survey of the existing infrastructure and its critical components. This type of exhaustive survey has not yet been conducted in human and social services, especially in terms of services for children. Thus, there is not a solid understanding of the infrastructure that exists. Given the lack of a critical infrastructure sector for human services, Lavin asked for suggestions to strengthen the infrastructure and build the knowledge base.

Simpson said she learned from this workshop that social services and educational services via the school system are the first areas that people think of for disaster response. Schools may be designated shelters or used as hubs for distributing food to families. However, these systems are already overtaxed, so when disaster strikes, they will have to implement continuity-of-operations plans. Therefore, the capabilities of other services in communities need to be built to support social and educational services. She stated that as a pediatrician, she is considering ways for her hospital system to conduct more targeted outreach to social services and to school systems in order to partner with the community to build the infrastructure needed to serve children.

Beal remarked that child care should be designated as critical infrastructure owing to its role in supporting recovery by simultaneously meeting the needs of children and enabling parents to work and rebuild. She added that currently, child care is often considered small business. She contended that as 60 percent of child care is for-profit, there is a large effect on communities when child care centers close. However, she remarked that there is no distinction between child care providers and other types of businesses in terms of grants, funding, and loan availability. Furthermore, there is no connection between child care and mental health support services. While these services are connected to schools, this access point is not available for younger children, she noted. Trauma and loss issues affect children of all ages, so greater support is needed for these services, whether or not they are classified as businesses.

Lavin quoted the statistic that of the 3,896,000 child care settings in the United States, 3,767,000 are in homes (Child Trends, 2020). Therefore, the child care facilities that most people envision only account for 129,000 settings across the country, making it all the more difficult to conceptualize child care as infrastructure. She contrasted this with banks, which are considered critical infrastructure. Somers noted that many times when people think of infrastructure, they think of physical space. For example, when people envision banks, they may think of physical locations and ATMs rather than of the services banks provide.

When considering the infrastructure needs of child care settings, early education, and schools, many people likely think of characteristics such as buildings having functioning water and electrical services. Somers noted that the services aspect of infrastructure is more abstract and should be conceptualized more holistically to encompass both physical space and services. Amler added that the COVID-19 pandemic has severely affected the state of New York, with quarantines undercutting people's ability to work and meet their own needs, and creating an increase in needs to be addressed by human services. Much can be learned from the pandemic and applied to other disaster-related events, she suggested. Lavin noted that programs discussed at this workshop, such as the children and youth task force in Puerto Rico, psychological first aid, and child care disaster planning requirements can be learned from and replicated.

Beal remarked that a human services sector needs to be built in which child care is defined as critical infrastructure. Child care includes tangible structures, such as child care centers and schools, in addition to the services it offers. She noted that the current critical infrastructure sectors do not cover child care buildings and services or mental health services. Amler suggested that sometimes the unmet needs of children seem so large that adequately addressing them is perceived as an impossible task. Improvements should be approached piece by piece, starting small and building up. Rather than attempting to overhaul the system all at once, addressing individual pieces can be successful and make the task less daunting, she added.

Simpson said she approaches issues through her health care system lens, where clinical conditions are addressed by examining the evidence base of data and research that applies to different populations in treating a particular illness. Referencing information on evidence gaps presented at this conference, Simpson noted that data are needed to measure the effectiveness of model programs being built at the local level. Many efforts to mitigate the effects of disasters on children are not yet present in the literature. Additional data would allow communities to learn from one another and would provide a benchmark of best practices for various situations and for different age groups of children and their adult supports.

Lori Peek, director of the Natural Hazards Center and professor at the University of Colorado Boulder, referenced a book, *Palaces for the People: How Social Infrastructure Can Help Fight Inequality, Polarization, and the Decline of Civic Life*, which argues that the physical infrastructure of schools, parks, libraries, and child care supports social infrastructure (Klinenberg, 2018). Lavin contended that first addressing the critical infrastructure of human services would likely enable other issues to be addressed, such as supporting service providers and building capacity of voluntary organizations active in disaster, and thus better meet the needs of children during a disaster.

Initiatives and Actions with Greatest Potential Effect

Lavin asked what initiatives or actionable items might have the most effect moving forward. Beal highlighted the value of using children and youth task forces, but she noted that this particular structure may not be applicable to every area owing to a lack of resources to organize it. Furthermore, task forces would look different in various locations, as membership, design, and leadership will vary. However, Beal said that incorporating processes such as children's task forces into standard emergency management planning efforts would place greater emphasis on children's needs. Rather than considering children's needs at the end of planning efforts, children's needs and resources should be identified ahead of time so that gaps can be resolved before disasters take place.

Simpson pointed out that many programs currently exist that have been built on the lessons learned from Hurricane Katrina, but technical assistance may be needed in order for communities to access these programs. Thus, it is not only a matter of establishing services, but also of creating better systems of connecting programs and the people most in need. Programs also need to be operationalized so that the outcomes of services can be measured, thus enabling them to be built on each time new lessons are learned from a disaster, she added.

Responding to a participant's comment that advocates should demand that emergency management systems in their local communities address the needs of children, Lavin said that access to resources will be required to scale up and integrate services for children. A single organization such as Save the Children (STC) cannot cover all child-related disaster needs. More engagement is needed, beginning with emergency management systems and establishing a larger leadership role for human services and agencies such as the Administration for Children and Families (ACF). Lavin said that in large-scale disasters, both bottom-up and top-down approaches are needed.

Amler emphasized that children should not be an afterthought: children are the future and should be the first population considered, not the last. The typical approach is planning for everyone else, and then making considerations for children and those with special needs—this paradigm should be flipped. She suggested that by addressing the most difficult considerations at the front end, populations with fewer needs would simultaneously be covered. Lavin added that a utilitarian approach of "the greatest good for the greatest number" results in serving "the wealthy and the healthy," to the exclusion of everyone else.

In considering actions that might be most promising or have the greatest effect, Lavin said that a top priority is accessibility of data. A plethora of data has been generated, but the people who are able to take large amounts of data and distill them down into evidence generally lack access to data on disaster interventions. Another priority is addressing issues arising from school closings, such as the effect this has on food insecurity, she said. Additionally, she suggested effecting policy changes, such as the emergent electronic benefits transfer and advancing benefits before an imminent disaster.

Beal pointed out many providers of child care and child-related services lack a clear understanding of the Small Business Administration (SBA) loan process. In her dissertation research on Superstorm Sandy, she found that providers were not aware that they could apply for these loans. Although SBA makes this information available, it would be helpful if additional organizations assisted in making child care providers aware of their options regarding SBA loans before a disaster hits. For instance, child care professionalization organizations, state licensing groups, and ACF could offer more training and information on how to navigate the SBA system, she suggested.

To reduce silos and broaden perspectives, Somers suggested that entities and organizations should reach out across sectors and professions. In her work around environmental health at the Agency for Toxic Substances and Disease Registry, Somers has collaborated with ACF regarding children's exposures to environmental contaminants after disasters. Such collaborations lead to thinking about problems and issues in a new way. Once working relationships are established across professions, organizations become information resources for one another. For example, in her work in environmental health, Somers can reach out to colleagues in early child care and education when she is approaching an issue involving children. Child care, education, environmental health, and mental health are all important needs, so breaking down the barriers between silos to share data and best practices with one another improves the work of each profession.

Supporting Children and Youth in School Settings

Given that children spend much of their day in school settings, Lavin asked how schools can be better used to provide disaster-related education of teachers and students—and perhaps of community members and volunteers as well. Amler suggested that regular education around disaster preparedness be taught in schools, beginning in kindergarten. Children should be taught what to do in disaster situations and take an active part in disaster-related drills, for example. She added that in public health, much time is spent drilling on processes (e.g., points of distribution), but the pediatric population is rarely included in the actual drills. She suggested that children's active participation in a variety of disaster-related drills would decrease their anxiety should an event occur; it would also provide them with the knowledge of what to do in such situations. For example, teaching children cardiopulmonary resuscitation (CPR) or how to dial 911 enables them to know what to do in an emergency.

Given that children in the child welfare system have predisaster vulnerability, Lavin asked how predisaster conditions can be accounted for in disaster response and recovery. Amler commented that adverse childhood experiences (ACEs) are relevant in this context. That is, the trauma experienced by many children in the child welfare system puts them at a greater risk for both health-related and mental health conditions, which can decrease their ability to cope in a disaster-related event. She suggested that foster parents and people sponsoring children should be trained to have a fundamental understanding of disaster preparedness and a basic plan in place for managing an emergency event while the child is in their care. Simpson added that a community understanding of the natural grief reaction is lacking in the general population. Regardless of ACEs or predisposing conditions, Simpson said there is a need to learn "the 'CPR' for the grief response of tragedy and coping," because this would help people to cope before their needs rise to the level of requiring specialized mental health services or behavioral health specialists. The capacity of adults to understand and support children in an evidence-based way can be expanded through psychological first aid and other systems that are known to work in communities, Simpson suggested. Somers remarked that at this unique time in history of heightened discussion of equity and justice, the timing may be right to better understand the specific vulnerabilities of communities and populations, especially those of children.

Monitoring and Evaluation of Support Efforts

Lavin asked about strategies to monitor and evaluate the performance of disaster response and recovery efforts as they relate to human and social services. One strategy would be to fund disaster research specific to human services and encourage researchers to use available ACF data for assessment. Citing the need for holistic approaches that include government agencies, she asked the panel how interventions can be monitored and evaluated in order to generate evidence and in turn have evidence-based programs and responses. Amler said that it is best to look at lessons learned after events have occurred to determine what worked and what did not work. She noted that this approach is not theoretical, and that data are often readily available. Although it is not a hurricane or natural disaster, COVID-19 presents similar issues and provides an opportunity to learn how systems function and whether the most vulnerable families can be supported. In examining the response to any type of disaster, it becomes evident where the holes are, Amler stated.

Simpson said there are benefits to community-based participatory research. Noting that many organizations are developing systems and resources serving the same populations, she suggested that organizations share experiences and collect data from families experiencing multiple parts of the system simultaneously. Breaking down silos allows health care, social services, and other community programs to work together not only to develop programs but also to share in the evaluation process. Data building and collection can enable organizations to learn lessons together in real time, she added. For example, when she has a project in the emergency room, she can extend this to talking to school systems, case management systems, and so forth as she builds out her projects.

Lavin asked how government agencies could approach the evaluation of evidence collected about prevention interventions designed for children in schools. Somers responded by saying that federal agencies could aggregate the best practices they have observed and make them available to the public, which would empower local community members with knowledge about how to rebuild their communities. Organizations such as ACF, STC, and the American Red Cross can be sources of good information for community members, she added.

Lavin stated that while many people of higher socioeconomic status think of child care as private, for-profit facilities, the majority of providers that ACF helps to support are not-for-profit and serve some of the most financially disadvantaged people in the country, as is the case with many other social supports and human services organizations. Indeed, many of these not-for-profit organizations rely on volunteers. Lavin pointed out that data collection and evaluation efforts are far more feasible for large corporations than for small, not-for-profit organizations who do not have the staff capacity to conduct these activities.

Closing reflections called for strengthening child care infrastructure, placing the needs of children in the center of disaster preparation efforts, increasing resource and data accessibility, supporting interdisciplinary collaboration including considerations of the impact of trauma, better educating children about disaster preparedness, and monitoring and evaluating response and recovery efforts.

References

Abramson, D. M., T. Stehling-Ariza, Y. S. Park, L. Walsh, and D. Culp. 2010. Measuring individual disaster recovery: A socioecological framework. *Disaster Medicine and Public Health Preparedness* 4(Suppl 1):S46–S54. https://www.ncbi.nlm.nih.gov/pubmed/23105035 (accessed December 18, 2020).

Anderson, W. A. 2005. Bringing children into focus on the social science disaster research agenda. *International Journal of Mass Emergencies and Disasters* 23(3):159–175. http://ijmed.org/articles/376/download (accessed December 18, 2020).

Bagwell, H. B., R. Liggin, T. Thompson, K. Lyle, A. Anthony, M. Baltz, M. Melguizo-Castro, T. Nick, and D. Z. Kuo. 2016. Disaster preparedness in families with children with special health care needs. *Clinical Pediatrics* 55(11):1036–1043. https://www.ncbi.nlm.nih.gov/pubmed/27630005 (accessed December 18, 2020).

Baker, L. R., and M. D. Baker. 2010. Disaster preparedness among families of children with special health care needs. *Disaster Medicine and Public Health Preparedness* 4(3):240–245. https://www.ncbi.nlm.nih.gov/pubmed/21149221 (accessed December 18, 2020).

Baker, L. R., and L. A. Cormier. 2013. Disaster preparedness and families of children with special needs: A geographic comparison. *Journal of Community Health* 38(1):106–112. https://www.ncbi.nlm.nih.gov/pubmed/22821052 (accessed December 18, 2020).

Boon, H., L. Brown, and P. Pagliano. 2014. Emergency planning for students with disabilities: A survey of Australian schools. *Australian Journal of Emergency Management* 29:45–49.

Boustan, L. P., M. E. Kahn, P. W. Rhode, and M. L. Yanguas. 2020. The effect of natural disasters on economic activity in US counties: A century of data. *Journal of Urban Economics* 118:103257. http://www.sciencedirect.com/science/article/pii/S0094119020300280 (accessed December 18, 2020).

Child Trends. 2020. *Most child care settings in the United States are homes, not centers.* https://www.childtrends.org/most-child-care-providers-in-the-united-states-are-based-in-homes-not-centers (accessed December 18, 2020).

DHS (Department of Homeland Security). 2006. *The federal response to Hurricane Katrina: Lessons learned.* http://library.stmarytx.edu/acadlib/edocs/katrinawh.pdf (accessed December 18, 2020).

Fifolt, M., J. Wakelee, L. Eldridge Auffant, R. Carpenter, and L. Hites. 2017. Addressing the needs of adults and children with disabilities through emergency preparedness and organizational improvisation. *Nonprofit Management and Leadership* 27(3):423–434.

Fothergill, A., and L. A. Peek. 2015. *Children of Katrina.* https://utpress.utexas.edu/books/fothergill-peek-children-of-katrina (accessed May 6, 2021).

Grolnick, W. S., D. J. Schonfeld, M. Schreiber, J. Cohen, V. Cole, L. Jaycox, J. Lochman, B. Pfefferbaum, K. Ruggiero, K. Wells, M. Wong, and D. Zatzick. 2018. Improving adjustment and resilience in children following a disaster: Addressing research challenges. *American Psychology* 73(3):215–229. https://www.ncbi.nlm.nih.gov/pubmed/29446960 (accessed December 18, 2020).

Haeffele, S., and V. H. Storr. 2020. *Bottom-up responses to crisis.* London, UK: Palgrave MacMillan.

Hipper, T. J., R. Davis, P. M. Massey, R. M. Turchi, K. M. Lubell, L. E. Pechta, D. A. Rose, A. Wolkin, L. Briseno, J. L. Franks, and E. Chernak. 2018. The disaster information needs of families of children with special healthcare needs: A scoping review. *Health Security* 16(3):178–192. https://www.ncbi.nlm.nih.gov/pubmed/29883200 (accessed December 18, 2020).

HRSA (Health Resources and Services Administration) Maternal & Child Health Bureau. 2020. *Children and youth with special health care needs.* https://mchb.hrsa.gov/maternal-child-health-topics/children-and-youth-special-health-needs#2 (accessed December 18, 2020).

International Federation of Red Cross and Red Crescent Societies. 2007. *World disasters report.* Geneva, Switzerland: International Federation of Red Cross and Red Crescent Societies.

Klinenberg, E. 2018. *Palaces for the people: How social infrastructure can help fight inequality, polarization, and the decline of civic life*: New York: Broadway Books.

Lavin, R., C. Revere, and T. Veenema. 2009. *National Commission on Children and Disasters interim report.* https://training.fema.gov/hiedu/docs/public%20sector%20incident%20response%20-%20national%20commission%20on%20children%20in%20disasters%20report.pdf (accessed December 18, 2020).

McAdams Ducy, E., and L. M. Stough. 2011. Exploring the support role of special education teachers after Hurricane Ike: Children with significant disabilities. *Journal of Family Issues* 32(10):1325–1345.

Mohammad, L., and L. A. Peek. 2019. Exposure outliers: Children, mothers, and cumulative disaster exposure in Louisiana. *Journal of Family Strengths* 19(1).

NCCD and AHRQ (National Commission on Children and Disasters and Agency for Healthcare Research and Quality). 2010. *2010 report to the president and Congress.* http://purl.fdlp.gov/GPO/gpo3907 (accessed December 18, 2020).

Peek, L. 2008. Children and disasters: Understanding vulnerability, developing capacities, and promoting resilience—an introduction. *Children, Youth and Environments* 18(1):1–29. https://www.jstor.org/stable/10.7721/chilyoutenvi.18.1.0001 (accessed December 18, 2020).

Peek, L., and S. Domingue. 2020. Recognizing vulnerability and capacity: Federal initiatives focused on children and youth across the disaster life cycle. In *Government responses to crisis*, edited by S. Haeffelle and V. Storr. London, UK: Palgrave MacMillan. Pp. 61–87.

Peek, L., and L. M. Stough. 2010. Children with disabilities in the context of disaster: A social vulnerability perspective. *Child Development* 81(4):1260–1270. https://www.ncbi.nlm.nih.gov/pubmed/20636694 (accessed December 18, 2020).

Ronoh, S., J. Gaillard, and J. Marlowe. 2015a. Children with disabilities and disaster risk reduction: A review. *International Journal of Disaster Risk Science* 6(1):38–48.

Ronoh, S., J. C. Gaillard, and J. Marlowe. 2015b. Children with disabilities and disaster preparedness: A case study of Christchurch. *Kōtuitui: New Zealand Journal of Social Sciences Online* 10(2):91–102. https://doi.org/10.1080/1177083X.2015.1068185 (accessed December 18, 2020).

Steffen, S. L., and A. Fothergill. 2019. 9/11 volunteerism: A pathway to personal healing and community engagement. *Social Science Journal* 46(1):29–46.

Stough, L. M., and I. Kelman. 2018. People with disabilities and disasters. In *Handbook of disaster research*, edited by H. Rodriguez, E. Quarantelli, and R. Dynes. New York: Springer. Pp. 225–242.

Stough, L. M., E. M. Ducy, and D. Kang. 2017. Addressing the needs of children with disabilities experiencing disaster or terrorism. *Current Psychiatry Reports* 19(4):24. https://www.ncbi.nlm.nih.gov/pubmed/28405894 (accessed December 18, 2020).

Stough, L. M., E. M. Ducy, D. Kang, and S. Lee. 2020. Disasters, schools, and children: Disability at the intersection. *International Journal of Disaster Risk Reduction* 45:101447.

Weber, L., and L. A. Peek. 2014. *Displaced: Life in the Katrina diaspora*. Austin, TX: The University of Texas Press.

Wolf-Fordham, S., C. Curtin, M. Maslin, L. Bandini, and C. D. Hamad. 2015. Emergency preparedness of families of children with developmental disabilities: What public health and safety emergency planners need to know. *Journal of Emergency Management* 13(1):7.

Appendix A

Workshop Statement of Task

At the request of the Administration for Children and Families, the National Academies of Sciences, Engineering, and Medicine will conduct a series of three meetings exploring promising practices, ongoing challenges, and potential opportunities since Hurricane Katrina in the coordinated delivery of human and social services service programs following federally declared major natural disasters.

Each workshop will focus on a different emerging topic within disaster human services. Topic areas identified for each workshop are:

1. Children and youth in disasters;
2. Populations displaced by disaster; and
3. Data and information sharing for disaster human services.

Specific attention will focus on populations operating at a predisaster socioeconomic deficit and/or currently receiving government support services.

All workshops will include discussions of disaster response coordination and transition to reconstitution of routine service delivery programs by state, local, tribal, and territorial social services, human services, and public health agencies. Participants will also discuss current practices for the assessment and evaluation of outcomes from the aforementioned service delivery transition.

An appointed ad-hoc committee will plan each of three workshops. The committee will develop the agenda for each workshop session, select and invite speakers and discussants, and moderate the discussions. In accordance with institutional guidelines, designated rapporteurs will prepare proceedings of each workshop based on the presentations and discussions during that workshop. Following the conclusion of all three workshops, the designated rapporteurs will prepare a proceedings-in-brief as a high-level summary of the entire series. The proceedings will be subject to appropriate review procedures before release.

Appendix B

Workshop Agenda

From Hurricane Katrina to Paradise Wildfires: Exploring Themes in
Disaster Human Services:
A Workshop Series

July 22–23, 2020

WORKSHOP OBJECTIVES

- Understand the critical child infrastructure (i.e., the existing systems and networks of human and social services that serve children and youth) and how it functions (i.e., how services are delivered) before, during, and after a major federally declared natural or environmental disaster
- Understand the impact of disasters on children and youth that benefit from human and social services providers
- Understand the current gaps and future opportunities for supporting the coordinated delivery during and the restoration of services following a major federally declared natural disaster
- Explore potential matrices for evaluating response and recovery efforts related to human and social services

Day 1, July 22, 2020

10:00 AM   Chairs' Welcome
Aim: Orient participants to the space and the workshop

>   **Roberta Lavin**
>   Professor, College of Nursing, University of New Mexico
>   Workshop Planning Committee Chair

10:05 AM   Sponsor's Charge
Aims:
- *Present rationale for the workshop*
- *Review the Administration for Children and Families' (ACF's) goals during and after disasters*

>   *Presenters:*
>   **Scott M. Lekan**
>   Principal Deputy Assistant Secretary
>   ACF, Department of Health and Human Services (HHS)
>
>   **Natalie Grant**
>   Director, Office of Human Services Emergency Preparedness and Response
>   ACF, HHS

10:30 AM   Panel I: Critical Child Infrastructure
Aims:
- *Review existing systems and networks of social and human services that serve children and how they are delivered before a major federally declared disaster*
- *Identify flaws and gaps in steady states that are only more harmful when disaster strikes*

>   *Moderator:*
>   **Tarah Somers**
>   Regional Director, Region 1
>   Agency for Toxic Substances and Disease Registry
>
>   *Discussants:*
>   **Josephine Bias-Robinson**
>   Board Member
>   Life Pieces to Masterpieces

APPENDIX B

    Deborah Bergeron
    Director, Office of Head Start and Early Childhood Development
    ACF, HHS

11:15 AM   Break

11:30 AM   **Panel II: Impact of Disasters on Critical Child Infrastructure**
Aims:
- *How are the systems/networks of social and human services that serve children and youth affected during and after a major federally declared natural or environmental disaster?*
- *How are the services delivered during and after a disaster?*

    Moderator:
    Robert Amler
    Dean and Professor of Public Health
    New York Medical College

    Discussants:
    Trevor Riggen
    Senior Vice President, Disaster Cycle Services
    American Red Cross

    Lauralee Koziol
    National Advisor on Children and Disasters
    Federal Emergency Management Agency, Department of Homeland Security

    David Markenson
    Director and Medical Director
    Center of Excellence in Precision Responses to Bioterrorism and Disasters, New York Medical College

    Shannon Christian
    Director, Office of Child Care
    ACF, HHS

    Madeline Sullivan
    Office of Safe and Supportive Schools, Department of Education

12:30 PM   Lunch Break

1:00 PM   Case Studies—Impact of Disasters of Specific Populations
Aims:
- Highlight the experiences/needs of children/youth with issues brought on by or exacerbated by disasters
- Highlight provider/service challenges/best practices for specific subpopulations of children, youth, and families

Moderator:
Joelle Simpson
Medical Director of Emergency Preparedness
Children's National Health System

Discussants:
Scott Needle
Chief Medical Officer
Elica Health Center

Tara Powell
Associate Professor
University of Illinois at Urbana-Champaign

Merritt D. Schreiber
Department of Pediatrics
Lundquist Institute
Harbor-UCLA Medical Center
David Geffen School of Medicine, University of California, Los Angeles

Alice Fothergill
Professor of Sociology
The University of Vermont

Impact of Disasters on Parents and Guardians

Moderator:
Heather Beal
Founder and President
BLOCKS Inc.

Discussants:
Holly Nett
Director, Child Care Emergency Partnerships
Child Care Aware of America

Jonathan Sury
Project Director
National Center for Disaster Preparedness
Columbia University

C. J. Huff
Educator and Child Advocate

Impact of Disasters on Children with Complex or Special Needs

Moderator:
Ann-Marie Sabrsula
Education Coordinator
The Arc Westchester Children's School for Early Development

Discussants:
Laura Stough
Associate Professor
Assistant Director of the Center on Disability and Development
Texas A&M University

Carmen Sanchez
Education Program Specialist
Department of Education

Kate Moran
Education Program Specialist
Department of Education

Impact of Disasters on Unaccompanied Minors

Moderator:
Roberta Lavin
Professor, College of Nursing, University of New Mexico
Workshop Planning Committee Chair

Discussants:
Jeff Daniels
Program Manager, Runaway and Homeless Youth
ACF, HHS

Patricia Frost
Vice Chair
National Pediatric Disaster Coalition

Leanne McCallum
Task Force Coordinator
Greater New Orleans Human Trafficking Task Force

Joy E. Paluska
Program Manager in Disaster Preparedness and Response Program
National Center for Missing and Exploited Children

2:25 PM   Break

2:30 PM   Keynote: Exposure Outliers: Children Coming of Age in an Age of Environmental Extremes

Aims:
- *Describe the effects of childhood exposure to three or more major community disruptions*
- *Explain why we should mobilize as a community to prevent disasters*

Lori Peek
Professor, Department of Sociology
Director, Natural Hazards Center
University of Colorado Boulder

2:55 PM   Chair's Reflections and Preview of Day 2

Roberta Lavin
Professor, College of Nursing, University of New Mexico
Workshop Planning Committee Chair

3:00 PM   **ADJOURN**

APPENDIX B

Day 2, July 23, 2020

12:15 PM Welcome and Recap of Day One
Aims:
- *Orient participants to the workshop and the technology*
- *Recap Day 1*

> **Roberta Lavin**
> Professor, College of Nursing, University of New Mexico
> Workshop Planning Committee Chair

12:45 PM Panel III: Exploring the Gaps in Evidence
Aim: Deep dive into gaps in evidence

> *Moderator:*
> **Heather Beal**
> Founder and President
> BLOCKS Inc.
>
> *Discussants:*
> **Lori Peek**
> Professor, Department of Sociology
> Director, Natural Hazards Center
> University of Colorado Boulder
>
> **Amanda Rivera**
> Executive Director
> Youth Development Institute of Puerto Rico
>
> **David Schonfeld**
> Developmental-Behavioral Pediatrician and Professor of Clinical Pediatrics
> University of Southern California and Children's Hospital Los Angeles
>
> **Irwin Redlener**
> Clinical Professor
> Earth Institute, Columbia University

1:45 PM Break

1:55 PM   Planning Committee Reflections and Closing

Aims:
- *Understand the current gaps and future opportunities for supporting the coordinated delivery during, and the restoration of services following, a major federally declared natural disaster*
- *Explore potential matrices for evaluating response and recovery efforts related to social and human services*

> *Moderator:*
> **Roberta Lavin**
> Professor, College of Nursing, University of New Mexico
> Workshop Planning Committee Chair
>
> *Speakers:*
> **Sherlita Amler**
> Commissioner
> Westchester County, New York, Department of Health
>
> **Joelle Simpson**
> Medical Director of Emergency Preparedness
> Children's National Health System
>
> **Heather Beal**
> Founder and President
> BLOCKS Inc.
>
> **Tarah Somers**
> Regional Director, Region 1
> Agency for Toxic Substances and Disease Registry

2:40 PM   **ADJOURN**

Appendix C

Speaker Biographies

Robert Amler, M.D., M.B.A., is the dean of the School of Health Sciences and Practice at the New York Medical College and the vice president for government affairs. Dr. Amler was previously the regional health administrator at the Department of Health and Human Services, where he secured supplemental State Children's Health Insurance Program funding for Medicaid programs. He oversaw hospital emergency preparedness and directed federal medical emergency assets during heightened external threats to the region. As the chief medical officer at the Centers for Disease Control and Prevention's (CDC's) Agency for Toxic Substances and Disease Registry, he coordinated medical monitoring for anthrax response teams, launched a nationwide program to protect children from chemical hazards, established standardized environmental medicine biomarkers, and created a nationwide clinical network (Pediatric Environmental Health Specialty Units) that has since expanded to several other countries. A practicing physician, Dr. Amler is a graduate of Dartmouth College; New York University; Rutgers, The State University of New Jersey; the Robert Wood Johnson Medical School; and CDC's Epidemic Intelligence Service, with residencies at Bellevue Hospital and St. Luke's–Roosevelt Hospital.

Deborah Bergeron, Ph.D., M.Ed., is the director of the Office of Head Start (OHS). Known as "Dr. B" to former students and teachers, she has been a teacher at heart for her entire life and has spent three decades in pre-K–12 public education as a classroom teacher and elementary and high school administrator. In the course of her career, Dr. Bergeron also started, grew, and ultimately sold her own educational services company. During her tenure as a school administrator, she specialized in school improvement. In three different school systems, Dr. Bergeron used strategies around school climate and effective instruction to inspire staff. In turn, staff were able to provide students with programming and instruction that yielded significant gains, including reading, math, discipline, and graduation rates. Since joining OHS in April 2018, Dr. Bergeron has used her experience as an elementary principal and her strong background in pre-K–12 instructional leadership to provide unique insights into how Head Start can support the most vulnerable children to become school ready. She has focused her energy on improving the relationship between Head Start and the public school system and continues to work at both the national level and with education influencers at the state and local levels to affect change. In January 2019, Dr. Bergeron was asked to broaden her leadership to include the Office of Early Childhood Development (ECD) in the Administration for Children and Families. Her vision for ECD in conjunction with the work for OHS is to transform how the nation prioritizes early childhood programming and to create a more collaborative, cohesive environment for early childhood. Dr. Bergeron holds a bachelor's degree from Texas State University. She earned a master's in education leadership and a doctorate in education policy from George Mason University.

Josephine Bias-Robinson is an executive leader with more than 20 years of organization transformation, life cycle communications, and people strategy expertise. She has led strategic relationships, national partnerships, and campaigns across multiple sectors and industries including education, workforce, health care, and financial services. Her focus is always to bring organizations closer to the people they serve. Most recently she served as the executive vice president of external affairs for the HSC Health Care System (HSC), a subacute special health care system dedicated to serving children and youth with chronic medical conditions and disabilities. She came to HSC after serving as the chief of family and public engagement for the District of Columbia Public Schools (DCPS). As part of the Chancellor's Management Team, her partnership work with families and community stakeholders improved family engagement and helped move DCPS to become one of the fastest rising school systems in the nation. Prior to her work at DCPS, Ms. Bias-Robinson served as the vice president for financial stability and community impact for United Way Worldwide and in various roles at the Department of Health and Human Services and the White House, including the director of community services at the Administration for Children and Families, the associate director of the White House Office of Public Liaison, and an executive assistant to the chief of staff to President George W. Bush. Committed to matters related to children and families, she has served on numerous local boards focused on children and youth.

Shannon Christian, M.P.P., serves as the director of the Office of Child Care at the Department of Health and Human Services' (HHS's) Administration for Children and Families (ACF). She is a former associate commissioner of the former Child Care Bureau at ACF, where she advanced President George W. Bush's Good Start, Grow Smart early childhood initiative, and shaped the office's research agenda to better support state policy and spending decisions. Committed to effective prevention strategies, Ms. Christian oversaw the launch of Illinois' home visiting program and was an active board member of Be Strong Families, a Chicago-based national nonprofit organization. Earlier in her career, Ms. Christian was part of former Wisconsin Governor (and HHS secretary) Tommy Thompson's welfare reform team, serving as the head of the planning section in the state Health and Social Services Department's Office of Policy and Budget, and as the senior advisor to the secretary of workforce development. Ms. Christian has an M.P.P. from the Harvard Kennedy School of Government, a certificate in nonprofit management from the Northwestern University Kellogg School of Business, and an undergraduate degree in economics and international relations from California State University, Chico.

Jeff Daniels is the regional program manager in Regions VIII, IX, and X for the Runaway and Homeless Youth (RHY) program at the Family and Youth Services Bureau in the Denver Regional Office. Mr. Daniels has more than 22 years of leadership, management, and administrative experience in government, including the Department of Defense, with expertise in leadership development, strategic planning, RHY program partnership, policy development, grant management, budget oversight, and congressional finance. He has held leadership positions as the Family Service Center director, Community Service Center director, Youth Program director, and commanding officer of a Transition Team. In his previous position while serving on active duty in the Marine Corps, he was responsible for all fiscal, administrative, and management duties for an agency with a budget in excess of $14 million annually. He led and supervised more than 50 military and civilian personnel in a seven-state region encompassing the southwestern United States. Additionally, while serving as the Transition Team commanding officer, he worked with the Iraqi government establishing runaway and homeless shelters, emergency clinics, and training procedures for more than 100 personnel. He has a B.S. in government and an M.S. in human development from Texas A&M University along with an M.B.A. from Webster University.

Alice Fothergill, Ph.D., is a professor of sociology at The University of Vermont (UVM). She studies disasters, children, inequality, and vulnerability. She and co-researcher Lori Peek conducted a longitudinal study on the experiences of children and youth in Hurricane Katrina, which resulted in the 2015 award-winning book *Children of Katrina*. Professor Fothergill is an editor of *Social Vulnerability to Disasters*, first and second editions. Her book *Heads Above Water: Gender, Class, and Family in the Grand Forks Flood* examines women's experiences in the 1997 flood in Grand Forks, North Dakota. Following the September 11, 2001, terrorist attacks, Professor Fothergill and her co-researcher Dr. Seana Lowe Steffen studied volunteerism in New York City, exploring how volunteers were affected by their efforts in the short and long term. In the aftermath of Tropical Storm Irene in 2011, she took her UVM sociology of disaster students into devastated Vermont communities to help with recovery efforts for a unique community-based, service-learning experience. In 2017, Professor Fothergill was a Fulbright Fellow in New Zealand, examining disaster preparedness in child care centers. Originally from Washington, DC, she was a research associate at the Natural Hazards Center at the University of Colorado, and then a faculty member at the University of Akron in Ohio, before joining the Department of Sociology at UVM in 2003. Presently, she is embarking on a 2-year study of children and the elderly in the COVID-19 pandemic.

Patricia Frost, RN, M.S.N., PHN, PNP, is the vice chair for the National Pediatric Disaster Coalition and recently retired as the director of emergency medical services for Contra Costa County in California. Ms. Frost received her B.S.N. from the University of San Francisco in 1977, her M.S.N. in 1983, and her post-master's Pediatric Nurse Practitioner in 1995 from the University of California, San Francisco. Ms. Frost has an extensive background as a pediatric clinician in prehospital, inpatient, ambulatory, and critical care settings, serving in a variety of roles including nurse practitioner, clinical educator, and nurse, and has served on medical missions in Ecuador and Vietnam. Ms. Frost is currently the education project manager for the Eastern Great Lakes Pediatric Consortium for Disaster Response and serves as an adjunct faculty member for the Federal Emergency Management Agency's Mgt. 439 Pediatric Disaster Response and Emergency Preparedness Course.

Natalie Grant, M.P.H., joined the Department of Health and Human Services' (HHS's) Administration for Children and Families as the director of the Office of Human Services Emergency Preparedness and Response (OHSEPR) in November 2018. In this capacity, she oversees the disaster human service emergency management mission for the agency and the department. OHSEPR's primary responsibilities include preparing human and social services programs and providers for disaster incidents; overseeing coordinated delivery of disaster human services case management; developing a disaster and applied science agenda for human services; supporting the coordination of support services for children, youth, and families in emergencies; and overseeing emergency repatriation mission for U.S. citizens overseas during international crises. Previously, she worked for HHS's Assistant Secretary for Preparedness and Response in the Division of Recovery, where she served as the Health and Social Services Recovery field coordinator for federal interagency coordination following Superstorm Sandy in New York and the lead for the U.S. Virgin Islands and Puerto Rico following Hurricanes Irma and Maria. She has also managed other disaster and emergency incidents within HHS Regions 1, 2, 5, and 10. Prior to her federal role, Ms. Grant served as the director of the Office of Public Health Preparedness at Boston Emergency Medical Services within the Boston Public Health Commission. She received her M.P.H. in international health from Boston University and A.B. in biology from Harvard College.

C. J. Huff, Ed.D., is an educator with more than 20 years of experience as a classroom teacher, building principal, and superintendent of schools. On May 22, 2011, the costliest tornado in U.S. history hit Joplin, Missouri. This EF-5 tornado with winds in excess of 200 mph devastated the community, killing 161 community members including 7 students and a staff member. As a school system, 10 of the 19 schools in his district were damaged or destroyed. Dr. Huff was responsible for successfully leading his district of 1,100 employees and 7,700 students through the community response and recovery effort that followed. Retiring from Joplin Schools in July 2015, Dr. Huff currently serves as a subject-matter expert to the Department of Health and Human Services and Louisiana State University, supporting preparedness, response, and recovery for natural and human-made disasters. In addition, he serves as an advisor to the national not-for-profit organizations Safe and Sound Schools and Bright Futures USA, working to build capacity and community resiliency to address the myriad of challenges facing children and youth across the nation.

Lauralee Koziol has led the Federal Emergency Management Agency's (FEMA's) efforts for nearly a decade to ensure that children's needs are integrated and implemented into disaster planning, preparedness, response, and recovery efforts starting at the federal level. This has been done by developing and institutionalizing tools and resources throughout FEMA and collaborating closely with federal, state, territorial, local, nongovernmental, and pediatric partners across the nation. In addition to her work on a national level, she has led field efforts to support children and their families in the aftermath of the Joplin, Moore, and El Reno tornadoes; Superstorm Sandy; Baton Rouge floods; and Hurricane Maria. She has served on the Department of Health and Human Services' National Advisory Committee on Children and Disasters, the Department of Homeland Security's Blue

Campaign to Combat Human Trafficking, and as a principal advisor during the 2014 Unaccompanied Alien Children Influx.

Scott Lekan, M.B.A., serves as the principal deputy assistant secretary and the acting commissioner of the Office of Child Support Enforcement (OCSE) in the Administration for Children and Families (ACF) within the Department of Health and Human Services. Mr. Lekan previously served as the assistant director of Arizona's Department of Economic Security. In that role, he focused on improving child support program performance through detailed analysis of caseload data and close attention to customer service. While there, he expanded the traditional enforcement toolkit to include fatherhood, employment, and diversionary services. Additionally, he worked in the area of economic security in the Division of Aging and Adult Services. Before joining the Trump administration as the OCSE commissioner, Mr. Lekan worked as a business development manager for Informatix, Inc., providing services for child support and other human services agencies around the country. As the principal deputy assistant secretary, Mr. Lekan serves as the chief operating officer of ACF and oversees both the Office of Regional Operations and the Office of Human Services Emergency Preparedness and Response. Additionally, he works to promote assistant secretary Johnson's goals, including a focus on primary prevention and economic mobility. Whether in human services, his 21-year career in law enforcement, or achieving his B.S. in criminal justice from Northern Arizona University and M.B.A. from California Pacific University, the keys to his success have been strong leadership, lean organization, and a passion for public service.

David Markenson, M.D., M.B.A., the director of the Center for Disaster Medicine at New York Medical College, co-founded the center in 2005 and is currently the medical director and a professor of public health. Dr. Markenson serves as the chief medical officer for training series, the chair of the National Scientific Advisory Council for the American Red Cross, and the chair of the Evidence-Based Group for Health for the International Federation of Red Cross and Red Crescent Societies. In addition to these roles, he serves as the deputy editor-in-chief for *Disaster Medicine and Public Health Preparedness*, the premier Medline indexed journal in the field of disaster medicine. Over the course of his extensive career in pediatrics, disaster medicine, emergency management, and public health, Dr. Markenson has become an internationally recognized expert in all aspects of disaster medicine, public health preparedness, and operational medicine with a unique expertise in the areas of pediatric considerations, health care planning and education, and planning for persons with disabilities. Dr. Markenson received his M.D. from the Albert Einstein College of

Medicine and his M.B.A. from the University of Massachusetts Amherst. Following medical school, Dr. Markenson completed his residency in general pediatrics followed by a pediatric chief resident year and fellowship training in both pediatric emergency medicine and pediatric critical care. His career has been dedicated to improving hospital and health system quality, improving the approach to pediatric care, disaster medicine and health care emergency management, and advancing emergency medical services and emergency medicine.

Leanne McCallum is the task force coordinator of the Greater New Orleans Human Trafficking Task Force. As the task force coordinator, she facilitates multidisciplinary collaboration among law enforcement, social services, and other sectors to enhance partnerships to combat human trafficking. Her work in the Greater New Orleans region centers on facilitating evidence-based, trauma-informed antitrafficking response. She has been featured as an expert speaker for a variety of local and national organizations, including the International Association of Chiefs of Police, the Bureau of Justice Assistance, the Office of Victims of Crime, and the HEAL Network. She began her interest in antitrafficking efforts as part of a collaborative ASIANetwork Freeman Foundation Fellowship, studying human trafficking of vulnerable populations in Southeast Asia. She earned her M.A. in international studies from the University of Denver Josef Korbel School of International Studies, graduating with concentrations in human rights and human trafficking. She received her undergraduate degree from Linfield College with a B.A. in international relations and a minor in political science.

Kate Moran, Ph.D., has dedicated her life to the education of students who have learning disabilities, mental challenges, and other health impairments. For more than 12 years, Dr. Moran has overseen States Special Education programs at the Department of Education's Office of Special Education Programs (OSEP). In addition to her role as a state lead, she has two lead areas, disaster response and private schools. In October 2017, after volunteering to participate in the Federal Emergency Management Agency (FEMA) Surge Capacity Force, she was deployed to Puerto Rico for 45 days, assisting Hurricane Irma and Hurricane Maria survivors through an assignment to the Disability Integration Team on the western side of the island, in Mayagüez. The work experience with FEMA has proven invaluable to her work at OSEP. In December 2014, she received her doctorate in special education leadership from George Mason University, and she has worked in the field of education for more than 25 years. Dr. Moran's research focused on the effects of the CrossFit Kids Program on improved academics and fitness with students with disabilities. Dr. Moran studied theater at The Catholic

University of America and followed that with a master's in special education from the University of Virginia. After graduation she ran a behavior program with Loudoun County Public Schools, Virginia, and was a special education coordinator with Alexandria City Public Schools, Virginia, prior to obtaining her position at the Department of Education.

Scott Needle, M.D., is the chief medical officer and a practicing community pediatrician for Elica Health Centers, a federally qualified health center in Sacramento, California. He serves on the Executive Committee of the American Academy of Pediatrics' (AAP's) Council on Children and Disasters. Prior to this he was a member of AAP's Disaster Preparedness Advisory Council from its inception in 2007 until 2019. Dr. Needle also served as the chair of the Department of Health and Human Services' National Advisory Committee on Children and Disasters from 2017 to 2018. He has written and lectured extensively on the needs of children and the role of pediatricians in disaster preparedness, response, and recovery, and he has worked closely with numerous local, state, and federal groups. He was one of the lead authors on the 2015 AAP policy statement "Ensuring the Health of Children in Disasters." Previous work with the Centers for Disease Control and Prevention includes helping to develop guidance on Zika, anthrax, and pandemic influenza. Dr. Needle received his M.D. from the Johns Hopkins University School of Medicine in Baltimore and completed his pediatric internship and residency at the New England Medical Center/Tufts University in Boston.

Holly Nett serves as the director of child care emergency partnerships at Child Care Aware of America. She has a primary focus on bridging the gap between the emergency preparedness, response, and recovery industry and child care programs. She also develops and delivers emergency preparedness training and technical assistance to child care resource and referral teams and child care program staff across the nation. This training and assistance is focused on business continuity, disaster plan development, and helping children and caregivers deal with the social and emotional aftermath of a disaster. Her professional service includes more than 20 years of experience in the child care resource and referral industry within the states of North Dakota and Minnesota, where she held leadership roles focused primarily on coaching and technical assistance systems development and delivery for early childhood programs. Ms. Nett has a B.S. in child development and family science from North Dakota State University.

Joy Paluska joined the National Center for Missing and Exploited Children in 2019 as a program manager in the Missing Children Division. In this role, she oversees the Disaster Preparedness and Response Program and supports special projects related to children on the autism spectrum and children of color. Between 2010 and 2018, Ms. Paluska served as a civil servant within the Executive Office of the President. Prior to that she worked in disaster recovery with both the Federal Emergency Management Agency and the American Red Cross. Ms. Paluska began her career at the Leadership Conference on Civil and Human Rights and following that, worked as an attorney for Legal Aid and in private practice in her home state of Illinois. Ms. Paluska is a graduate of The University of Iowa and The City University of New York School of Law at Queens College.

Lori Peek, Ph.D., is the director of the Natural Hazards Center and a professor in the Department of Sociology at the University of Colorado Boulder. She is a co-author of *Children of Katrina*, the author of *Behind the Backlash: Muslim Americans After 9/11*, and a co-editor of *Displaced: Life in the Katrina Diaspora*. Dr. Peek helped create the Federal Emergency Management Agency's P-1000, *Safer, Stronger, Smarter: A Guide to Improving School Natural Hazard Safety*, which is the first comprehensive, natural hazards–focused school safety guidance for the nation. In addition to her work on potentially vulnerable populations in disaster, Dr. Peek is also the leader of the National Science Foundation–supported CONVERGE facility, the Social Science Extreme Events Research network, and the Interdisciplinary Science and Engineering Extreme Events Research network.

Tara Powell, Ph.D.'s research explores the impact of postdisaster behavioral health interventions in disaster-affected communities throughout the United States and internationally. She began her career as a clinical social worker in New Orleans after Hurricane Katrina. As both a hurricane survivor and postdisaster service provider, Dr. Powell recognized the need for behavioral health programs to address and prevent the emotional toll of a collective trauma such as Hurricane Katrina. Most recently she has examined the effect of community-based mental health interventions for Syrian refugees in Jordan, and with health care providers after Hurricanes Harvey and Maria. She also has been responding to the COVID-19 pandemic, providing webinars on self-care, supporting distressed children and youth, and helping with grief and bereavement. She provides expertise in stress management and coping skills, psychoeducational curriculum development, and aiding children, families, and communities after a collective trauma.

Trevor Riggen, M.P.P., was appointed as the senior vice president for Disaster Cycle Services at the American Red Cross (ARC) on January 2, 2019. In this role, Mr. Riggen leads a team of ARC staff and volunteer experts in disaster preparedness, response, and recovery. Team members develop and implement programs and conduct operations aimed at preventing and alleviating human suffering in the face of emergencies within the United States and its territories. Prior to this, Mr. Riggen served as the chief executive officer of the Northern California Coastal Region, where he provided management oversight of ARC services and supported a team of more than 7,000 volunteers and employees who responded to more than 800 local disasters each year and served more than 8 million residents with lifesaving programs. Prior to coming to ARC, Mr. Riggen held several leadership positions with community-based organizations in Illinois and in the Washington, DC, metro area. These positions focused on literacy, crime prevention, poverty reduction, education, and emergency planning for public school districts. He also served in the Peace Corps in Morocco, where he developed local agricultural cooperatives. Mr. Riggen earned his B.S. in political science from the University of Illinois and an M.P.P. from Georgetown University.

Amanda Rivera, M.P.P., is the executive director of the Youth Development Institute (YDI), Puerto Rico's only entity strictly dedicated to research, policy, and advocacy around children's issues, with a particular focus on child poverty. She is a leader committed to providing opportunities so that all children and youth in Puerto Rico can develop to their full potential. From being a middle school teacher through the Teach for America program to the director of development and community relations in a school in Harlem, New York, to leading federal policy efforts around child welfare and youth mental health, she has more than 15 years of experience working for children and youth and promoting public policy and education research. She worked as a public policy associate at edCount in Washington, DC, where she served as the assistant director of the Department of Education of Puerto Rico's Technical Assistance Project, and authored studies on the cognitive validity of standardized tests and school culture. Prior to YDI, she also led all federal policy efforts for Youth Villages, a nonprofit organization that serves 23,000 young people and their families in 13 states. Additionally, she is the co-founder of Puerto Rican Minds in Action (Mentes Puertorriqueñas en Acción), an entity with a mission to empower a network of young agents of change to create inclusive and effective initiatives for Puerto Rico. She has a bachelor's degree in government and sociology from Harvard College, where she conducted her thesis on the implementation of the Special Communities Program in Puerto Rico and focused her studies on the issues of inequality and poverty on the island. She also received an M.P.P. from the Harvard Kennedy School of Government with a specialization in social and public policy and a focus on childhood and youth issues.

Ann-Marie Sabrsula has more than 25 years of experience working in the field of developmental disabilities, with a specialization in young children (from birth to age 5) with autism spectrum disorder. She is the current education coordinator and co-administrator for the Arc Westchester Children's School for Early Development. Ms. Sabrsula earned her master's degree in applied developmental psychology and postgraduate work in school-building leadership, and she has presented on various topics related to early childhood special education and young children with developmental disabilities for community-based programs, school districts, local early intervention councils, and in support of the professional development of early intervention and preschool educational staff as well as family-focused trainings and workshops.

Carmen Sánchez is an education program specialist in the Office of Special Education Programs at the Department of Education, serving as the lead for the parent training and information center program for families of children with disabilities throughout the country. In addition, she is the project officer for the Center for Parent Information and Resources and the Center on Alternative Dispute Resolution in Special Education. Ms. Sánchez has also worked for local government, providing information and referral on disability issues across the life span.

David Schonfeld, M.D., FAAP, established and directs the National Center for School Crisis and Bereavement (www.schoolcrisiscenter.org) located at Children's Hospital Los Angeles. He is a professor of clinical pediatrics at the Keck School of Medicine. Prior faculty positions have been in the Department of Pediatrics at the Yale University School of Medicine, the head of the Section of Developmental and Behavioral Pediatrics at Cincinnati Children's Hospital Medical Center, the pediatrician-in-chief at St. Christopher's Hospital for Children, and the chair of pediatrics at the Drexel University College of Medicine. For more than 30 years, he has provided consultation and training to schools on supporting students and staff at times of crisis and loss in the aftermath of numerous school crisis events and disasters within the United States and abroad, including the COVID-19 pandemic (2020); terrorist attacks of the World Trade Center (2001); school and community shootings and stabbings in Santa Clarita, California (2019), Parkland, Florida (2018), Newtown, Connecticut (2012), Benton, Kentucky (2018), Las Vegas, Nevada (2017), Thousand Oaks, California (2018), Floresville, Texas (Sutherland Springs church) (2017), Marysville, Washington (2014), Osaka, Japan (2001), Corning, California (2017), Aurora, Colorado (2012), Platte Canyon, Colorado (2006), Chardon, Ohio (2012), and Townville, South Carolina (2016); flooding from Hurricane Maria in San Juan, Puerto Rico (2017), Superstorm Sandy in New York and New Jersey (2012), Hurricane Katrina in New Orleans, Louisiana (2005), and Hurricane Ike in Galveston, Texas (2008); tornadoes in Joplin, Missouri

(2011), and Alabama (2011); wildfires in Butte County, California (2018), Sonoma County, California (2017), and in the Great Smoky Mountains in Sevierville, Tennessee (2016); and the 8.0-magnitude earthquake in Sichuan, China (2008). Dr. Schonfeld is a member of the Executive Committee of the American Academy of Pediatrics Council on Disaster Preparedness and Recovery (formerly the Disaster Preparedness Advisory Council) and the National Biodefense Science Board. He served as a commissioner for both the National Commission on Children and Disasters and the Sandy Hook Advisory Commission in Connecticut. He served as the president of the Society for Developmental and Behavioral Pediatrics from 2006 to 2007.

Merritt D. Schreiber, M.D., is a professor of clinical pediatrics in the Department of Pediatrics at the Harbor-UCLA Medical Center, the Lundquist Research Institute, and the David Geffen School of Medicine at the University of California, Los Angeles. He leads the mental health working group for the University of California, San Francisco, Pediatric Disaster Medical Center of Excellence. Dr. Schreiber created the PsySTART Rapid Mental Health Triage Incident Management System for stepped triage to care via rapid identification of at-risk victims and emergency responders. PsySTART has been used throughout the United States and internationally. He is also the developer of "Anticipate, Plan, and Deter," a disaster medical provider triage and resilience system. Dr. Schreiber has actively deployed to multiple mass casualty events for adults, children, and first responders, including the American Red Cross–led Family Assistance Centers for AA 11, 77, and United 173 at Los Angeles International Airport after 9/11. He deployed for the National Disaster Medical System and the Public Health Service Commissioned Corps as a reserve officer to Hurricane Katrina, with the Centers for Disease Control and Prevention for the Southeast Tsunami, and most recently he deployed for the National Disaster Medical System for the COVID-19 Quarantine at Marine Corps Air Station Miramar.

Laura Stough, Ph.D., is the assistant director at the Center on Disability and Development, an associate professor of educational psychology, and a faculty fellow at the Hazards Reduction and Recovery Center at Texas A&M University. Dr. Stough's research investigates how environmental hazards affect individuals with disabilities and other historically marginalized populations. She is the co-author of *Disaster and Disability: Explorations and Exchanges*, which includes 19 chapters written by individuals with disabilities from around the world on their experiences with disasters and emergencies. Dr. Stough serves as the chair of the Disability Task Force for the Division on Emergency Management for the State of Texas and the chair of the Special Interest Group on Emergency Preparedness for the Association of University Centers on Disabilities.

Madeline Sullivan is a management and program analyst in the Department of Education's Office of Safe and Healthy Students. She also serves as the contracting officer's representative for the Readiness and Emergency Management for Schools Technical Assistance Center. Prior to joining the federal government workforce, she provided technical assistance on prosocial skill development, violence prevention, and school emergency management after having served as a special educator.

Jonathan Sury, M.P.H., is the project director for communications and field operations at the National Center for Disaster Preparedness (NCDP). He holds an M.P.H. in environmental health sciences with a concentration in environment and molecular epidemiology from the Columbia University Mailman School of Public Health. He has a keen interest in geographic information systems and their use in disaster preparedness and recovery. Presently, he contributes to a variety of disaster-related research at NCDP, including community resilience and child-focused preparedness, evaluating the unanticipated consequences of pandemic flu, determining racially and ethnically appropriate emergency messaging, analyzing the long-term disaster resiliency and recovery issues in the Gulf Coast following Hurricane Katrina, and the measurement and mapping of social vulnerability and the role of place and space in disaster recovery.